DIABETIC MEAL PREP

FOR BEGINNERS

500+ Delicious & Comfort Recipes For A Healthy Lifestyle
With 30-Day Diet Meal Plan

Sarah R. Wooten

Table of Contents

INTRODUCTION

Fighting diabetes is a lifetime commitment. Even if your blood glucose levels have normalized, it does not mean that you can go back to an idle lifestyle and eat the wrong foods. Slacking will surely bring back the symptoms. However, if you commit to doing aerobic exercises and a diabetes-friendly eating program for at least 30 days, it will jumpstart your path towards healthy living for the rest of your life.

Remember it only takes 30 days to commit to this and you can change your health forever. Just commit to two things for the following 30 days: 30 minutes of exercise every day and eating only your choice of diabetic-friendly meals for 30 days.

You should also check your progress regularly to ensure you are doing things right. Eating healthy foods and exercising for the following 30 days will surely make you look and feel a lot better. However, if you are a diabetic, you cannot base the evidence that your health is getting better merely on whether you gained weight, lost weight or look healthier. Blood sugar levels constantly need to be checked.

This is a small handy digital unit that you can easily buy in a pharmacy. A sterile needle (lancet) is used to prick the tip of a finger to draw a drop of blood to be placed in the test strip. The strip is then inserted in the digital device and will read the blood glucose level within just a few seconds. Blood is drawn out of the fingertips because it is the area in the body that reacts fastest to changes in glucose levels.

There are also different types of glucose monitoring devices that can test the forearms, thighs, the base of the thumb and the upper arm. For diabetics, blood glucose levels should ideally be checked several times throughout the day. Some check it every time they feel symptoms kicking in such as cravings, frequent urinations or extreme sleepiness after consuming a meal.

The type of doctor you should be seeing if you happen to have diabetes is an Endocrinologist because they have a special training in treating people with diabetes. However, to ensure complete overall care, there should be a team of doctors and experts you should be visiting regularly who can help you manage various symptoms. These include a primary care doctor, a dietician, an eye doctor, a dentist, a podiatrist, a physical trainer, and a diabetes educator.

BREAKFAST RECIPES

1. Granola with Fruits

Preparation Time: 15 minutes
Cooking Time: 35 minutes
Servings: 6
Ingredients:

- 3 cups quick cooking oats
- 1 cup almonds, sliced
- ½ cup wheat germ
- 3 tablespoons butter
- 1 teaspoon ground cinnamon
- 1 cup honey
- 3 cups whole grain cereal flakes
- ½ cup raisins
- ½ cup dried cranberries
- ½ cup dates, pitted and chopped

Directions:

1. Preheat your oven to 325 degrees F.
2. Place the almonds on a baking sheet.
3. Bake for 15 minutes.
4. Mix the wheat germ, butter, cinnamon and honey in a bowl.
5. Add the toasted almonds and oats.
6. Mix well.
7. Spread on the baking sheet.
8. Bake for 20 minutes.
9. Mix with the rest of the ingredients.
10. Let cool and serve.

Nutrition: Calories 210 Total Fat 7 g Saturated Fat 2 g Cholesterol 5 mg Sodium 58 mg Total Carbohydrate 36 g Dietary Fiber 4 g Total Sugars 2 g Protein 5 g Potassium 250 mg

2. Apple & Cinnamon Pancake

Preparation Time: 15 minutes
Cooking Time: 10 minutes
Servings: 4
Ingredients:

- ¼ teaspoon ground cinnamon
- 1 ¾ cups Better Baking Mix
- 1 tablespoon oil
- 1 cup water
- 2 egg whites
- ½ cup sugar-free applesauce
- Cooking spray
- 1 cup plain yogurt
- Sugar substitute

Directions:

1. Blend the cinnamon and the baking mix in a bowl.
2. Create a hole in the middle and add the oil, water, egg and applesauce.
3. Mix well.
4. Spray your pan with oil.
5. Place it on medium heat.
6. Pour ¼ cup of the batter.
7. Flip the pancake and cook until golden.

8. Serve with yogurt and sugar substitute.

Nutrition: Calories 231 Total Fat 6 g Saturated Fat 1 g Cholesterol 54 mg Sodium 545 mg Total Carbohydrate 37 g Dietary Fiber 4 g Total Sugars 1 g Protein 8 g Potassium 750 mg

3. Spinach Scramble

Preparation Time: 5 minutes
Cooking Time: 15 minutes
Servings: 2
Ingredients:

- ¼ cup liquid egg substitute
- ¼ cup skim milk
- Salt and pepper to taste
- 2 tablespoons crumbled bacon
- 13 ½ oz. canned spinach, drained
- Cooking spray

Directions:

1. Mix the Ingredients in a large bowl.
2. Transfer the mixture on a pan greased with oil, placed over medium heat.
3. Stir until fully cooked.

Nutrition: Calories 70 Total Fat 2 g Saturated Fat 1 g Cholesterol 25 mg Sodium 700 mg Total Carbohydrate 5 g Dietary Fiber 2 g Total Sugars 1 g Protein 8 g Potassium 564 mg

4. Breakfast Parfait

Preparation Time: 5 minutes
Cooking Time: 0 minute
Servings: 2
Ingredients:

- 4 oz. unsweetened applesauce
- 6 oz. non-fat and sugar-free vanilla yogurt
- ¼ teaspoon pumpkin pie spice
- ¼ teaspoon honey
- 1 cup low-fat granola

Directions:

1. Mix the Ingredients except the granola in a bowl.
2. Layer the mixture with the granola in a cup.
3. Refrigerate before serving.

Nutrition: Calories 287 Total Fat 3 g Saturated Fat 1 g Cholesterol 28 mg Sodium 186 mg Total Carbohydrate 57 g Dietary Fiber 4 g Total Sugars 2 g Protein 8 g Potassium 4

5. Asparagus & Cheese Omelet

Preparation Time: 10 minutes
Cooking Time: 10 minutes
Servings: 2
Ingredients:

- Cooking spray
- 4 spears asparagus, sliced
- Pepper to taste
- 3 egg whites
- ½ teaspoon olive oil
- 1 oz. spreadable cheese, sliced
- 1 teaspoon parsley, chopped

Directions:

1. Spray oil on your pan.
2. Cook asparagus on the pan over medium high heat for 5 to 7 minutes.
3. Wrap with foil and set aside.
4. In a bowl, mix pepper and egg whites.
5. Add olive oil to the pan.
6. Add the egg whites.
7. When you start to see the sides forming, add the asparagus and cheese on top.
8. Sprinkle parsley on top before serving.

Nutrition: Calories 119 Total Fat 5 g Saturated Fat 2 g Cholesterol 10 mg Sodium 427 mg Total Carbohydrate 5 g Dietary Fiber 2 g Total Sugars 3 g Protein 15 g Potassium 308 mg

6. Sausage, Egg & Potatoes

Preparation Time: 15 minutes
Cooking Time: 10 hours and 10 minutes
Servings: 6
Ingredients:

- Cooking spray
- 12 oz. chicken sausage links, sliced
- 1 onion, sliced into wedges
- 2 red sweet peppers, sliced into strips
- 1 ½ lb. potatoes, sliced into strips
- ¼ cup low-sodium chicken broth
- Black pepper to taste
- ½ teaspoon dried thyme, crushed
- 6 eggs
- ½ cup low-fat cheddar cheese, shredded

Directions:

1. Spray oil on a heavy foil sheet.
2. Put the sausage, onion, sweet peppers and potatoes on the foil.
3. Drizzle top with the chicken broth.
4. Season with the pepper and thyme.
5. Fold to seal.
6. Place the packet inside a cooker.
7. Cook on low setting for 10 hours.
8. Meanwhile, boil the egg until fully cooked.
9. Serve eggs with the sausage mixture.

Nutrition: Calories 281 Total Fat 12 g Saturated Fat 4 g Cholesterol 262 mg Sodium 485 mg Total Carbohydrate 23 g Dietary Fiber 3 g Total Sugars 3 g Protein 21 g Potassium 262 mg

7. Cucumber & Yogurt

Preparation Time: 5 minutes
Cooking Time: 0 minute
Servings: 1
Ingredients:

- 1 cup low-fat yogurt
- ½ cup cucumber, diced
- ¼ teaspoon lemon zest
- ¼ teaspoon lemon juice
- ¼ teaspoon fresh mint, chopped
- Salt to taste

Directions:

1. Mix all the Ingredients in a jar.

2. Refrigerate and serve.

Nutrition: Calories 164 Total Fat 4 g Saturated Fat 2 g Cholesterol 15 mg Sodium 318 mg Total Carbohydrate 19 g Dietary Fiber 1 g Total Sugars 18 g Protein 13 g Potassium 683 mg

8. Yogurt Breakfast Pudding

Preparation Time: 8 hours and 10 minutes
Cooking Time: 0 minute
Servings: 2
Ingredients:

- ½ cup rolled oats
- 6 oz. low-fat yogurt
- ¼ cup canned pineapple
- ½ cup fat-free milk
- ½ teaspoon vanilla
- ⅛ teaspoon ground cinnamon
- 1 tablespoon flaxseed meal
- 4 teaspoons almonds, toasted and sliced
- ½ cup apple, chopped

Directions:

1. In a bowl, mix all the Ingredients except almonds and apple.
2. Transfer the mixture into an airtight container.
3. Cover with the lid and refrigerate for 8 hours.
4. Top with the almonds and apple before serving.

Nutrition: Calories 255 Total Fat 7 g Saturated Fat 1 g Cholesterol 5 mg Sodium 84 mg Total Carbohydrate 38 g Dietary Fiber 5 g Total Sugars 21 g Protein 11 g Potassium 345 mg

9. Vegetable Omelet

Preparation Time: 5 minutes
Cooking Time: 25 minutes
Servings: 4
Ingredients:

- ½ cup yellow summer squash, chopped
- ½ cup canned diced tomatoes with herbs, drained
- ½ ripe avocado, pitted and chopped
- ½ cup cucumber, chopped
- 2 eggs
- 2 tablespoons water
- Salt and pepper to taste
- 1 teaspoon dried basil, crushed
- Cooking spray
- ¼ cup low-fat Monterey Jack cheese, shredded
- Chives, chopped

Directions:

1. In a bowl, mix the squash, tomatoes, avocado and cucumber.
2. In another bowl, mix the eggs, water, salt, pepper and basil.
3. Spray oil on a pan over medium heat.
4. Pour egg mixture on the pan.
5. Put the vegetable mixture on top of the egg.
6. Lift and fold.
7. Cook until the egg has set.
8. Sprinkle cheese and chives on top.

Nutrition: Calories 128 Total Fat 6 g Saturated Fat 2 g Cholesterol 97 mg Sodium 357 mg Total Carbohydrate 7 g Dietary Fiber 3 g Total Sugars 4 g Protein 12 g Potassium 341 mg

10. Almond & Berry Smoothie

Preparation Time: 10 minutes
Cooking Time: 0 minute
Servings: 1
Ingredients:

- ⅔ cup frozen raspberries
- ½ cup frozen banana, sliced
- ½ cup almond milk (unsweetened)
- 3 tablespoons almonds, sliced
- ¼ teaspoon ground cinnamon
- ⅛ teaspoon vanilla extract
- ¼ cup blueberries
- 1 tablespoon coconut flakes (unsweetened)

Directions:

1. Put the Ingredients in a blender except coconut flakes. Pulse until smooth.
2. Top with the coconut flakes before serving.

Nutrition: Calories 360 Total Fat 19 g Saturated Fat 3 g Cholesterol 0 mg Sodium 89 mg Total Carbohydrate 46 g Dietary Fiber 14 g Total Sugars 21 g Protein 9 g Potassium 736 mg

11. Banana & Spinach Smoothie Bowl

Preparation Time: 10 minutes
Cooking Time: 10 minutes
Servings: 3
Ingredients:

- 2 small ripe frozen bananas, peeled and sliced
- ½ cup frozen blueberries
- 1 cup frozen spinach
- 1 cup cauliflower
- 1½ scoops unsweetened vegan protein powder
- 3 tablespoons peanut butter
- 2 tablespoons hemp seeds
- 1 teaspoon maca powder
- 1 teaspoon spirulina
- 1 cup unsweetened coconut milk

Directions:

1. Put all ingredients in a high-speed blender, and pulse until creamy.
2. Pour into three serving bowls and serve immediately with your favorite topping.

Nutrition: Calories 400 Total Fat 22.3 g Saturated Fat 12 g Cholesterol 0 mg Sodium 216 mg Total Carbs 32.6 g Fiber 4.9 g Sugar 17.4 g Protein 20.2 g

12. Mixed Berries Smoothie Bowl

Preparation Time: 10 minutes
Cooking Time: 10 minutes
Servings: 2
Ingredients:

- 2 large frozen bananas, peeled and sliced
- 1 cup frozen mixed berries

- 1 scoop unsweetened vegan protein powder
- ¼ cup unsweetened coconut milk

Directions:

1. In a high-speed blender, place all ingredients and pulse until creamy.
2. Pour into two serving bowls and serve immediately with your favorite topping.

Nutrition: Calories 242 Total Fat 5.2 g Saturated Fat 3.9 g Cholesterol 0 mg Sodium 77 mg Total Carbs 38.6 g Fiber 5.6 g Sugar 21.1 g Protein 11.7 g

13. Bulgur Porridge

Preparation Time: 10 minutes
Cooking time: 15 minutes
Servings: 2
Ingredients:

- 2/3 cup unsweetened soy milk
- 1/3 cup bulgur, rinsed
- Pinch of salt
- 1 ripe banana, peeled and mashed
- 2 kiwis, peeled and sliced

Directions:

1. In a pan, add the soy milk, bulgur, and salt over medium-high heat and bring to a boil.
2. Adjust the heat to low and simmer for about 10 minutes.
3. Remove the pan of bulgur from heat and immediately, stir in the mashed banana.
4. Serve warm with the topping of kiwi slices.

Nutrition: Calories 223 Total Fat 2.3 g Saturated Fat 0.3 g Cholesterol 0 mg Sodium 126 mg Total Carbs 47.5 g Fiber 8.6 g Sugar 17.4 g Protein 7.1 g

14. Buckwheat Porridge

Preparation Time: 10 minutes
Cooking time: 15 minutes
Servings: 2
Ingredients:

- 1½ cups water
- 1 cup buckwheat groats, rinsed
- ¾ teaspoon vanilla extract
- ½ teaspoon ground cinnamon
- ¼ teaspoon salt
- 2 tablespoons maple syrup
- 1 ripe banana, peeled and mashed
- 1½ cups unsweetened soy milk
- 1 tablespoon peanut butter
- 1/3 cup fresh strawberries, hulled and chopped

Directions:

1. Place the water, buckwheat, vanilla extract, cinnamon, and salt in a pan and bring to a boil.
2. Now, adjust the heat to medium-low and simmer for about 6 minutes, stirring occasionally.
3. Stir in maple syrup, banana, and soy milk, and simmer, covered for about 6 minutes.
4. Remove the pan of porridge from heat and stir in peanut butter.
5. Serve warm with the topping of strawberry pieces.

Nutrition: Calories 453 Total Fat 9.4 g Saturated Fat 1.7 g Cholesterol 0 mg Sodium 374 mg Total Carbs 82.8 g Fiber 9.4 g Sugar 28.8 g Protein 16.2 g

15. Quinoa Porridge

Preparation Time: 10 minutes
Cooking time: 20 minutes
Servings: 2
Ingredients:

- 1 cup dry quinoa, rinsed
- 1½ cups unsweetened almond milk
- 1 teaspoon vanilla extract
- 1 teaspoon ground cinnamon
- 2 tablespoons maple syrup
- 4 tablespoons peanut butter
- ¼ cup fresh strawberries, hulled and chopped
- ¼ cup fresh blueberries

Directions:

1. In a small pan, place quinoa, almond milk, vanilla extract, and cinnamon over medium heat and bring to a boil.
2. Now, adjust the heat to low and simmer, covered for about 15 minutes or until all the liquid is absorbed.
3. Remove the pan of quinoa from heat and stir in maple syrup and peanut butter.
4. Serve warm with the topping of berries.

Nutrition: Calories 608 Total Fat 24 g Saturated Fat 4.2 g Cholesterol 0 mg Sodium 289 mg Total Carbs 81 g Fiber 10 g Sugar 17.9 g Protein 21.1 g

16. Pumpkin Oatmeal

Preparation Time: 10 minutes
Cooking time: 2 minutes
Servings: 2
Ingredients

- 2 cups hot water
- 1/3 cup pumpkin puree
- 1/3 cup rolled oats
- 2 tablespoons chia seeds
- 1 teaspoon cinnamon
- 1 teaspoon ground ginger
- ¼ teaspoon ground nutmeg
- 2 scoops unsweetened vanilla vegan protein powder
- 1 tablespoon maple syrup

Directions:

1. In a microwave-safe bowl, place water, pumpkin puree, oats, chia seeds, and spices and mix well.
2. Microwave on High for about 2 minutes.
3. Remove the bowl of oatmeal from the microwave and stir in the protein powder and maple syrup.
4. Serve immediately.

Nutrition: Calories 223 Total Fat 4.6 g Saturated Fat 0.5 g holesterol 0 mg Sodium 137 mg Total Carbs 28.7 g Fiber 5.8 g Sugar 9.5 g Protein 22.9 g

17. Oatmeal Blueberry Pancakes

Preparation Time: 10 minutes
Cooking time: 40 minutes
Servings: 4

Ingredients

- ½ cup rolled oats
- ½ cup unsweetened almond milk
- ¼ cup unsweetened applesauce
- ¼ cup unsweetened vegan protein powder
- ½ tablespoon flax meal
- 1 teaspoon baking powder
- ½ teaspoon vanilla extract
- ¼ teaspoon baking soda
- ¼ teaspoon ground cinnamon
- 1/8 teaspoon salt
- ½ cup fresh blueberries

Directions:

1. Place all ingredients (except for blueberries) in a food processor and pulse until smooth.
2. Transfer the mixture into a bowl and set aside for 5 minutes.
3. Gently, fold in blueberries.
4. Place a lightly greased medium skillet over medium heat until heated.
5. Place desired amount of the mixture and cook for about 3–5 minutes per side.
6. Repeat with the remaining mixture.
7. Serve warm.

Nutrition: Calories 105 Total Fat 1.8 g Saturated Fat 0.2 g Cholesterol 0 mg Sodium 204 mg Total Carbs 15.4 g Fiber 2.2 g Sugar 5.2 g Protein 8 g

18. Tempeh & Veggie Hash

Preparation Time: 15 minutes
Cooking time: 25 minutes
Servings: 3
Ingredients:

- 2½ cups sweet potato, peeled and cubed
- 1/3 cup red onion, chopped finely
- 1 cup tempeh, cubed
- 1 cup Brussels sprout, quartered
- 2 garlic cloves, minced
- ½ teaspoon ground cumin
- ½ teaspoon garlic powder
- Salt and ground black pepper, to taste
- 1½ cups fresh kale, tough ribs removed and chopped

Directions:

1. In a pan of the boiling water, add the sweet potato cubes and cook for about 8 minutes.
2. Drain the sweet potato cubes completely.
3. Heat the canola oil in a skillet over medium-high heat and sauté the onion for about 4–5 minutes.
4. Add in remaining ingredients (except for spinach) and cook for about 6–7 minutes, stirring occasionally.
5. Add cooked sweet potato and kale and cook for about 5 minutes, stirring twice.
6. Serve hot.

Nutrition: Calories 298 Total Fat 6.5 g Saturated Fat 1.3 g Cholesterol 0 mg Sodium 139 mg Total Carbs 48.2 g Fiber 7.6 g Sugar 12.1 g Protein 16 g

19. Tofu & Zucchini Muffins

Preparation Time: 15 minutes
Cooking time: 40 minutes
Servings: 6
Ingredients:

- 12 ounces extra-firm silken tofu, drained and pressed
- ¾ cup unsweetened soy milk
- 2 tablespoons canola oil
- 1 tablespoon apple cider vinegar
- 1 cup whole-wheat pastry flour
- ½ cup chickpea flour
- 1 teaspoon baking powder
- ½ teaspoon baking soda
- 1 teaspoon smoked paprika
- 1 teaspoon onion powder
- 1 teaspoon salt
- ½ cup zucchini, chopped
- ¼ cup fresh chives, minced

Directions:

1. Preheat your oven to 400°F.
2. Line a 12-cup muffin tin with paper liners.
3. In a bowl, place tofu and with a fork, mash until smooth.
4. In the bowl of tofu, add almond milk, oil, and vinegar, and mix until slightly smooth.
5. In a separate large bowl, add flours, baking powder, baking soda, spices, and salt, and mix well.
6. Transfer the mixture into muffin cups evenly.
7. Bake for approximately 35–40 minutes or until a toothpick inserted in the center comes out clean.
8. Remove the muffin tin from oven and place onto a wire rack to cool for about 10 minutes.
9. Carefully invert the muffins onto a platter and serve warm.

Nutrition: Calories 237 Total Fat 9 g Saturated Fat 1 g Cholesterol 0 mg Sodium 520 mg Total Carbs 2293.3 g Fiber 5.9 g Sugar 3.7 g Protein 11.1 g

20. Strawberry & Spinach Smoothie

Preparation Time: 10 minutes
Cooking Time: 15 minutes
Servings: 2
Ingredients:

- 1½ cups fresh strawberries, hulled and sliced
- 2 cups fresh baby spinach
- ½ cup fat-free plain Greek yogurt
- 1 cup unsweetened almond milk
- ¼ cup ice cubes

Directions:

1. In a high-speed blender, add all the ingredients and pulse until smooth.
2. Pour into serving glasses and serve immediately.

Nutrition: Calories 96 Total Fat 2.3 g Saturated Fat 0.2 g Cholesterol 1 mg Total Carbs 12.3 g Sugar 7.7 g Fiber 3.9 g Sodium 144 mg Potassium 428 mg Protein 8.1 g

21. Millet Porridge

Preparation Time: 10 minutes
Cooking Time: 25 minutes
Servings: 4
Ingredients:

- 1 cup millet, rinsed and drained
- Pinch of salt
- 3 cups water
- 2 tablespoons almonds, chopped finely
- 6-8 drops liquid stevia
- 1 cup unsweetened almond milk
- 2 tablespoons fresh blueberries

Directions:

1. In a nonstick pan, add the millet over medium-low heat and cook for about 3 minutes, stirring continuously.
2. Add the salt and water and stir to combine
3. Increase the heat to medium and bring to a boil.
4. Cook for about 15 minutes.
5. Stir in the almonds, stevia and almond milk and cook for 5 minutes.
6. Top with the blueberries and serve.

Nutrition: Calories 219 Total Fat 4.5 g Saturated Fat 0.6 g Cholesterol 0 mg Total Carbs 38.2 g Sugar 0.6 g Fiber 5 g Sodium 92 mg Potassium 1721 mg Protein 6.4 g

22. Bell Pepper Pancakes

Preparation Time: 15 minutes
Cooking Time: 8 minutes
Servings: 2
Ingredients:

- ½ cup chickpea flour
- ¼ teaspoon baking powder
- Pinch of sea salt
- Pinch of red pepper flakes, crushed
- ½ cup plus 2 tablespoons filtered water
- ¼ cup green bell peppers, seeded and chopped finely
- ¼ cup scallion, chopped finely
- 2 teaspoons olive oil

Directions:

1. In a bowl, mix together flour, baking powder, salt and red pepper flakes.
2. Add the water and mix until well combined.
3. Fold in bell pepper and scallion.
4. In a large frying pan, heat the oil over low heat.
5. Add half of the mixture and cook for about 1-2 minutes per side.
6. Repeat with the remaining mixture.
7. Serve warm.

Nutrition: Calories 232 Total Fat 7.8 g Saturated Fat 1 g Cholesterol 0 mg Total Carbs 32.7 g Sugar 6.4 g Fiber 9.3 g Sodium 132 mg Potassium 566 mg Protein 10 g

23. Sweet Potato Waffles

Preparation Time: 10 minutes
Cooking Time: 20 minutes
Servings: 2
Ingredients:

- 1 medium sweet potato, peeled, grated and squeezed
- 1 teaspoon fresh thyme, minced
- 1 teaspoon fresh rosemary, minced
- 1/8 teaspoon red pepper flakes, crushed
- Salt and ground black pepper, as required

Directions:
1. Preheat the waffle iron and then grease it.
2. In a large bowl, add all ingredients and mix till well combined.
3. Place half of the sweet potato mixture into preheated waffle iron and cook for about 8-10 minutes or until golden brown.
4. Repeat with the remaining mixture.
5. Serve warm.

Nutrition: Calories 72 Total Fat 0.3 g Saturated Fat 0.1 g Cholesterol 0 mg Total Carbs 16.3 g Sugar 4.9 g Fiber 3 g Sodium 28 mg Potassium 369 mg Protein 1.6 g

24. Quinoa Bread

Preparation Time: 10 minutes
Cooking Time: 1½ hours
Servings: 12
Ingredients:

- 1¾ cups uncooked quinoa, rinsed, soaked overnight and drained
- ¼ cup chia seeds, soaked in ½ cup of water overnight
- ½ teaspoon bicarbonate soda
- Pinch of sea salt
- ½ cup filtered water
- ¼ cup olive oil, melted
- 1 tablespoon fresh lemon juice

Directions:
1. Preheat the oven to 320 degrees F. Line a loaf pan with a parchment paper.
2. In a food processor, add all the ingredients and pulse for about 3 minutes.
3. Transfer the mixture into loaf pan evenly.
4. Bake for about 1 hour.
5. Remove the pan from oven and place onto a wire rack to cool for about 10-15 minutes.
6. Carefully, remove the bread from the loaf pan and place onto the wire rack to cool completely before slicing.
7. With a sharp knife, cut the bread loaf into desired sized slices and serve.

Nutrition: Calories 137 Total Fat 6.5 g Saturated Fat 0.9 g Cholesterol 0 mg Total Carbs 16.9 g Sugar 0 g Fiber 2.6 g Sodium 203 mg Potassium 158 mg Protein 4 g

25. Tofu Scramble

Preparation Time: 15 minutes
Cooking Time: 15 minutes
Servings: 2
Ingredients:

- ½ tablespoon olive oil
- 1 small onion, chopped finely
- red bell pepper, seeded and chopped finely
- 1 cup cherry tomatoes, chopped finely

- 1½ cups firm tofu, pressed and crumbled
- Pinch of ground turmeric
- Pinch of cayenne pepper
- 1 tablespoon fresh parsley, chopped

Directions:
1. Heat the oil over medium heat
2. Cook bell pepper and the onion for about 4-5 minute.
3. Add the tomatoes and cook for about 1-2 minutes.
4. Add the tofu, turmeric and cayenne pepper and cook for about 6-8 minutes.
5. Garnish with parsley and serve.

Nutrition: Calories 213 Total Fat 11.8 g Saturated Fat 2.2 g Cholesterol 0 mg Total Carbs 14.7 g Sugar 8 g Fiber 4.5 g Sodium 31 mg Potassium 872 mg Protein 17.3 g

26. Apple Omelet

Preparation Time: 10 minutes
Cooking Time: 10 minutes
Servings: 3
Ingredients:

- 4 teaspoons olive oil, divided
- 2 small green apples, cored and sliced thinly
- ¼ teaspoon ground cinnamon
- Pinch of ground cloves
- Pinch of ground nutmeg
- 4 large eggs
- ¼ teaspoon organic vanilla extract
- Pinch of salt

Directions:
1. over medium-low heat in frying pan, heat 1 teaspoon
2. Place the apple slices and sprinkle with spices.
3. Cook for about 4-5 minutes, flipping once halfway through.
4. Meanwhile, in a bowl, add the eggs, vanilla extract and salt and beat until fluffy.
5. Add the remaining oil in the pan and let it heat completely.
6. Place the egg mixture over apple slices evenly and cook for about 3-5 minutes or until desired doneness.
7. Carefully, turn the pan over a serving plate and immediately, fold the omelet.
8. Serve immediately.

Nutrition: Calories 228 Total Fat 13.2 g Saturated Fat 3 g Cholesterol 248 mg Total Carbs 21.3 g Sugar 16.1 g Fiber 3.8 g Sodium 145 mg Potassium 251 mg Protein 8.8 g

27. Veggie Frittata

Preparation Time: 15 minutes
Cooking Time: 25 minutes
Servings: 6
Ingredients:

- 1 tablespoon olive oil
- 1 large sweet potato, cut and peeled into thin slices
- 1 yellow squash, sliced
- 1 zucchini, sliced
- ½ of red bell pepper, seeded and sliced

- ½ of yellow bell pepper, seeded and sliced
- 8 eggs
- Salt and ground black pepper, as required
- 2 tablespoons fresh cilantro, chopped finely

Directions:
1. Preheat the oven to broiler.
2. over medium-low heat, cook the sweet potato for about 6-7 minutes.
3. Add the yellow squash, zucchini and bell peppers and cook for about 3-4 minutes.
4. Meanwhile, in a bowl, add the eggs, salt and black pepper and beat until well combined.
5. Pour egg mixture over vegetables mixture.
6. Transfer the skillet in the oven and broil for about 3-4 minutes or until top becomes golden brown.
7. With a sharp knife, cut the frittata in desired size slices and serve with the garnishing of cilantro.

Nutrition: Calories 143 Total Fat 8.4 g Saturated Fat 2.2 g Cholesterol 218 mg Total Carbs 9.3 g Sugar 4.2 g Fiber 1.1 g Sodium 98 mg Potassium 408 mg Protein 8.9 g

28. **Chicken & Sweet Potato Hash**
Preparation Time: 15 minutes
Cooking Time: 35 minutes
Servings: 8
Ingredients:

- 2 tablespoons olive oil, divided
- 1½ pounds boneless, skinless chicken breasts, cubed
- Salt and ground black pepper, as required
- 2 celery stalks, chopped
- 1 medium white onion, chopped
- 4 garlic cloves, minced
- 1 tablespoon fresh oregano, chopped
- 1 tablespoon fresh thyme, chopped
- 2 large sweet potatoes, peeled and cubed
- 1 cup low-sodium chicken broth
- 1 cup scallion, chopped
- 2 tablespoons fresh lime juice

Directions:
1. heat 1 tablespoon of oil over medium heat and cook the chicken with a little salt and black pepper for about 4-5 minutes.
2. Transfer the chicken into a bowl.
3. In the same skillet, heat the remaining oil over medium heat and sauté celery and onion for about 3-4 minutes.
4. Add the garlic and herbs and sauté for about 1 minute.
5. Add the sweet potato and cook for about 8-10 minutes.
6. Add the broth and cook for about 8-10 minutes.
7. Add the cooked chicken and scallion and cook for about 5 minutes.
8. Stir in lemon juice, salt and serve.

Nutrition: Calories 253 Total Fat 10 g Saturated Fat 2.3 g Cholesterol 76 mg Total Carbs 14 g Sugar 1.2 g Fiber 2.6 g Sodium 92 mg Potassium 597 mg Protein 26 g

29. **Pancakes**
Preparation Time: 5 minutes
Cooking Time: 10 minutes
Servings: 2
Ingredients:

- 2 tbsp coconut oil
- 1 tsp maple extract
- 2 tbsp cashew milk
- 2 eggs

Directions:
1. Add the oil to a skillet. Add a quarter-cup of the batter and fry until golden on each side. Continue adding the remaining batter.

Nutrition: 260 cal.23g fat 7g protein 3g carbs

30. **Breakfast Sandwich**
Preparation Time: 10 minutes
Cooking Time: 0 minutes
Servings: 2
Ingredients:

- 2 oz/60g cheddar cheese
- 1/6 oz/30g smoked ham
- 2 tbsp butter
- 4 eggs

Directions:
1. Fry all the eggs and sprinkle the pepper and salt on them.
2. Place an egg down as the sandwich base. Top with the ham and cheese and a drop or two of Tabasco.
3. Place the other egg on top and enjoy.

Nutrition: 600 cal.50g fat 12g protein 7g carbs.

31. **Egg Muffins**
Preparation Time: 10 minutes
Cooking Time: 20 minutes
Servings: 6
Ingredients:

- 1 tbsp green pesto
- 3 oz/75g shredded cheese
- 5 oz/150g cooked bacon
- 1 scallion, chopped
- 6 eggs

Directions:
1. You should set your oven to 350°F/175°C.
2. Place liners in a regular cupcake tin. This will help with easy removal and storage.
3. Beat the eggs with pepper, salt, and the pesto. Mix in the cheese.
4. Pour the eggs into the cupcake tin and top with the bacon and scallion.
5. Cook for 15-20 minutes

Nutrition: 190 cal.15g fat 7g protein 4g carbs.

32. **Bacon & Eggs**
Preparation Time: 2 minutes
Cooking Time: 3 minutes
Servings: 4
Ingredients:

- Parsley
- Cherry tomatoes

- 5 1/3 oz/150g bacon
- 8 eggs

Directions:

1. Fry up the bacon and put it to the side.
2. Scramble the eggs in the bacon grease, with some pepper and salt. If you want, scramble in some cherry tomatoes. Sprinkle with some parsley and enjoy.

Nutrition: 80 cal 7g fat 14g protein 2g carbs.

33. Eggs on the Go

Preparation Time: 5 minutes
Cooking Time: 5 minutes
Servings: 4
Ingredients:

- 4 oz/110g bacon, cooked
- Pepper
- Salt
- 12 eggs

Directions:

1. You should set your oven to 200°C.
2. Place liners in a regular cupcake tin. This will help with easy removal and storage.
3. Crack an egg into each of the cups and sprinkle some bacon onto each of them. Season with some pepper and salt.
4. Bake for 15 minutes, or until the eggs are set.

Nutrition: 75 cal. 6g fat 8g protein 1g carbs.

34. Cream Cheese Pancakes

Preparation Time: 5 minutes
Cooking Time: 5 minutes
Servings: 1
Ingredients:

- 2 oz cream cheese
- 2 eggs
- ½ tsp cinnamon
- 1 tbsp keto coconut flour
- ½ to 1 packet of Stevia

Directions:

1. Skillet with butter the pan or coconut oil on medium-high.
2. Make them as you would normal pancakes.
3. Cook and flip one side to cook the other side!
4. Top with some butter and/or sugar-free syrup.

Nutrition: 340 cal.30g fat 7g protein 3g carbs

35. Breakfast Mix

Preparation Time: 10 minutes
Cooking Time: 5 minutes
Servings: 1
Ingredients:

- 5 tbsp coconut flakes, unsweetened
- 7 tbsp hemp seeds
- 5 tbsp flaxseed, ground
- 2 tbsp sesame, ground
- 2 tbsp cocoa, dark, unsweetened

Directions:

1. Grind the sesame and flaxseed.
2. only grind the sesame seeds for a small period..

3. Mix all ingredients in a jar and shake it well.
4. Keep refrigerated until ready to eat.
5. Serve softened with black coffee or even with still water and add coconut oil if you want to increase the fat content. It also blends well with cream or with mascarpone cheese.

Nutrition: 150 cal.9g fat 8g protein 4g carbs.

36. Breakfast Muffins

Preparation Time: 10 minutes
Cooking Time: 5 minutes
Servings: 1
Ingredients:

- 1 medium egg
- ¼ cup heavy cream
- 1 slice cooked bacon (cured, pan-fried, cooked)
- 1 oz cheddar cheese
- Salt and black pepper (to taste)

Directions:

1. Preheat the oven to 350°F.
2. In a bowl, mix the eggs with the cream, salt and pepper.
3. Spread into muffin tins and fill the cups half full.
4. Place 1 slice of bacon into each muffin hole and half ounce of cheese on top of each muffin.
5. Bake for around 15-20 minutes or until slightly browned.
6. Add another ½ oz of cheese onto each muffin and broil until the cheese is slightly browned. Serve!

Nutrition: 150 cal 11g fat 7g protein 2g carbs

37. Egg Porridge

Preparation Time: 10 minutes
Cooking Time: 10 minutes
Servings: 1
Ingredients:

- 2 organic free-range eggs
- 1/3 cup organic heavy cream without food additives
- 2 packages of your preferred sweetener
- 2 tbsp grass-fed butter ground organic cinnamon to taste

Directions:

1. In a bowl add the eggs, cream and sweetener, and mix together.
2. Melt the butter in a saucepan over a medium heat. Lower the heat once the butter is melted.
3. Combine together with the egg and cream mixture.
4. While Cooking, mix until it thickens and curdles.
5. When you see the first signs of curdling, remove the saucepan immediately from the heat.
6. Pour the porridge into a bowl. Sprinkle cinnamon on top and serve immediately.

Nutrition: 604 cal 45g fat 8g protein 2.8g carbs.

38. Eggs Florentine

Preparation Time: 10 minutes
Cooking Time: 10 minutes
Servings: 2
Ingredients:

- 1 cup washed, fresh spinach leaves

- 2 tbsp freshly grated parmesan cheese
- Sea salt and pepper
- 1 tbsp white vinegar
- 2 eggs

Directions:

1. Cook the spinach the microwave or steam until wilted.
2. Sprinkle with parmesan cheese and seasoning.
3. Slice into bite-size pieces
4. Simmer a pan of water and add the vinegar. Stir quickly with a spoon.
5. Break an egg into the center. Turn off the heat and cover until set.
6. Repeat with the second egg.
7. Place the eggs on top of the spinach and serve.

Nutrition: 180 cal.10g fat 7g protein 5g carbs.

39. Keto Creamy Bacon Dish

Preparation Time: 5 minutes
Cooking Time: 5 minutes
Servings: 2
Ingredients:

- ½ tsp dried basil
- ½ tsp minced garlic
- ½ tsp tomato paste
- 2 oz unsalted butter, softened
- 3 slices of bacon, chopped

Directions:

1. Bring out a skillet pan, put it over medium heat, add 1 tbsp butter and when it starts to melts, add chopped bacon and cook for 5 minutes.
2. Then remove the pan from heat, add remaining butter, along with basil and tomato paste, season with salt and black pepper and stir until well mixed.
3. Move bacon butter into an airtight container, cover with the lid, and refrigerate for 1 hour until solid.

Nutrition: 150 Cal 16 g Fats 1 g Protein 0.5 g Net Carb 1 g Fiber

40. Eggplant Omelet

Preparation Time: 10 minutes
Cooking Time: 5 minutes
Servings: 2
Ingredients:

- 1 large eggplant
- 1 tbsp coconut oil, melted
- 1 tsp unsalted butter
- 2 eggs
- 2 tbsp chopped green onions

Directions:

1. Set the grill and let it preheat at the high setting.
2. In the meantime, Prepare the eggplant, and for this, cut two slices from eggplant, about 1-inch thick, and reserve the remaining eggplant for later use.
3. Brush slices of eggplant with oil, season with salt on both sides, then Put the slices on grill and cook for 3 to 4 minutes per side.
4. Move grilled eggplant to a cutting board, let it cool for 5 minutes and then make a home in the center of each slice by using a cookie cutter.
5. Bring out a frying pan, put it over medium heat, add butter and when it melts, add eggplant slices in it and crack an egg into its each hole.
6. Let the eggs cook, then carefully flip the eggplant slice and continue cooking for 3 minutes until the egg has thoroughly cooked
7. Season egg with salt and black pepper, move them to a plate, then garnish with green onions and serve.

Nutrition: 184 Cal 14.1 g Fats 7.8 g Protein 3 g Net Carb 3.5 g Fiber

41. Keto Egg Scramble

Preparation Time: 2 minutes
Cooking Time: 3 minutes
Servings: 2
Ingredients:

- ¼ tsp salt
- 1 tbsp unsalted butter, softened
- 1/8 tsp ground black pepper
- 2 tbsp chopped unsalted butter, cold
- 3 eggs

Directions:

1. Bring out a bowl, cracked eggs in it, whisk until well combined, and then stir in chopped cold butter until mixed.
2. Bring out a skillet pan, put it over medium-low heat, add butter and when it melts, pour in the egg mixture and cook for 1 minute, don't stir.
3. Then stir the omelet and cook for 1 to 2 minutes until thoroughly cooked and scramble to the desired level.
4. Season scramble eggs with salt and black pepper and then serve.

Nutrition: 81.5 Cal 3.75 g Fats 3.75 g Protein 0.25 g Net Carb 0 g Fiber

42. Low Carb Pancakes and Cheese

Preparation Time: 2 minutes
Cooking Time: 3 minutes
Servings: 2
Ingredients:

- ½ tsp cinnamon
- 1 tsp unsalted butter
- 2 eggs
- 2 oz cream cheese

Directions:

1. Put cream cheese in a blender, add eggs and cinnamon, pulse for 1 minute or until smooth, and then let the batter rest for 5 minutes.
2. Bring out a skillet pan, put it over medium heat, add butter and when it melts, drop one-fourth of the batter into the pan, spread evenly, and cook the pancakes for 2 minutes per side until done.
3. Move pancakes to a plate and serve.

Nutrition: 97.8 Cal 8.4 g Fats 4.4 g Protein 1 g Net Carb 0.2 g Fiber

43. Egg-Veggie Scramble

Preparation Time: 2 minutes
Cooking Time: 3 minutes

Servings: 2
Ingredients:

- ¼ tsp salt
- 1 tbsp unsalted butter
- 1/8 tsp ground black pepper
- 3 eggs, beaten
- 4 oz spinach

Directions:

1. Bring out a frying pan, put it over medium heat, add butter and when it melts, add spinach and cook for 5 minutes until leaves have wilted.
2. Then pour in eggs, season with salt and black pepper, and cook for 3 minutes until eggs have scramble to the desired level.

Nutrition: 90 Cal 7 g Fats 5.6 g Protein; 0.7 g Net Carb 0.6 g Fiber

44. Egg "Dough" in a Pan

Preparation Time: 4 minutes
Cooking Time: 4 minutes
Servings: 2
Ingredients:

- ¼ tsp salt
- ½ of medium red bell pepper, chopped
- 1/8 tsp ground black pepper
- 2 eggs
- 2 tbsp chopped chives

Directions:

1. Turn on the oven, then set it to 350 degrees F and let it preheat.
2. In the meantime, crack eggs in a bowl, add remaining ingredients and whisk until combined.
3. Bring out a small heatproof dish, pour in egg mixture, and bake for 5 to 8 minutes until set.
4. When done, cut it into two squares and then serve.

Nutrition: 87 Cal 5.4 g Fats 7.2 g Protein 1.7 g Net Carb 0.7 g Fiber

45. Keto Low Carb Crepe

Preparation Time: 4 minutes
Cooking Time: 4 minutes
Servings: 2
Ingredients:

- 2 eggs
- 1 egg white
- 1 tbsp unsalted butter
- 1 1/3 tbsp cream cheese
- 2/3 tbsp psyllium husk

Directions:

1. Preparation the batter and for this, put all the ingredients in a bowl, except for butter, and then whisk by using a stick blender until smooth and very liquid.
2. Bring out a skillet pan, put it over medium heat, add ½ tbsp butter and when it melts, pour in half of the batter, spread evenly, and cook until the top has firmed.
3. Carefully flip the crepe, then continue cooking for 2 minutes until cooked and then move it to a plate.

4. Add remaining butter and when it melts, cook another crepe in the same manner and then serve.

Nutrition: 118 Cal 9.4 g Fats 6.5 g Protein 1 g Net Carb 0.9 g Fiber

46. Savory Keto Pancake

Preparation Time: 3 minutes
Cooking Time: 2 minutes
Servings: 2
Ingredients:

- ¼ cup almond flour
- 1 ½ tbsp unsalted butter
- 2 eggs
- 2 oz cream cheese, softened

Directions:

1. Bring out a bowl, crack eggs in it, whisk well until fluffy, and then whisk in flour and cream cheese until well combined.
2. Bring out a skillet pan, put it over medium heat, add butter and when it melts, drop pancake batter in four sections, spread it evenly, and cook for 2 minutes per side until brown.

Nutrition: 166.8 Cal 15 g Fats 5.8 g Protein 1.8 g Net Car 0.8 g Fiber

47. Mix Veggie Fritters

Preparation Time: 4 minutes
Cooking Time: 3 minutes
Servings: 2
Ingredients:

- ½ tsp nutritional yeast
- 1 oz chopped broccoli
- 1 zucchini, grated, squeezed
- 2 eggs
- 2 tbsp almond flour

Directions:

1. Wrap grated zucchini in a cheesecloth, twist it well to remove excess moisture, and then Put zucchini in a bowl.
2. Add remaining ingredients, except for oil, and then whisk well until combined.
3. Bring out a skillet pan, put it over medium heat, add oil and when hot, drop zucchini mixture in four portions, shape them into flat patties and cook for 4 minutes per side until thoroughly cooked.

Nutrition: 191 Cal 16.6 g Fats 9.6 g Protein 0.8 g Net Carb 0.2 g Fiber

48. Keto Cheese Rolls

Preparation Time: 5 minutes
Cooking Time: 0 minutes
Servings: 2
Ingredients:

- 1-oz butter, unsalted
- 2 oz mozzarella cheese, sliced, full-fat

Directions:

1. Cut cheese into slices and then cut butter into thin slices.
2. Top each cheese slice with a slice of butter, roll it and then serve.

Nutrition: 166 Cal 15 g Fats 6.5 g Protein 2 g Net Carb 0 g   Fiber

SIDE DISHES RECIPES

49. Creamed Coconut Curry Spinach

Preparation Time: 30 minutes
Cooking Time: 1 hr
Servings: 6
Ingredients:

- 1-pound frozen spinach, thawed and drained of moisture
- 1 small can whole fat coconut milk
- 2 tsp yellow curry paste
- 1 tsp lemon zest
- Cashews for garnish

Directions:

1. Heat a medium sized pan to medium high heat, then add the curry paste and cook for 30 seconds. Add a small amount of the coconut milk and stir to combine, then cook until the paste is aromatic.
2. Add the spinach, then season. Add the rest of the ingredients, apart from the cashews, and allow the sauce to reduce slightly.
3. Keep the sauce creamy, but reduce it to coat the spinach well. Serve with chopped cashews.

Nutrition: Net carbs: 3g, Protein: 4g, Fat: 18g, Calories: 191kcal.

50. Cauliflower Risotto

Preparation Time: 20 minutes
Cooking Time: 1 hr
Servings: 4
Ingredients:

- 4 cups riced raw cauliflower
- 2 tbsps. butter
- 1/2 tsp kosher salt
- 1/8 tsp black pepper
- 1/4 tsp garlic powder
- 1/3 cup mascarpone cheese
- 2 tbsps. parmesan cheese
- 1/4 cup premade basil pesto

Directions:

1. Mix everything but the cheeses and pesto in a microwavable bowl, then cook for 6-7 minutes on high, until the cauliflower is tender.
2. Mix the mascarpone cheese into the risotto and cook for 2 minutes. Mix well and season.
3. Fold the parmesan cheese into the risotto, until well incorporated. Add the pesto just before service, to preserve the green color. Serve hot.

Nutrition: Net carbs: 4g, Protein: 6g, Fat: 21g, Calories: 225kcal.

51. Garlic Chive Cauliflower Mash

Preparation Time: 20 minutes
Cooking Time: 1 hr
Servings: 5
Ingredients:

- 4 cups cauliflower
- 1/3 cup vegetarian mayonnaise
- 1 garlic clove
- 1/2 tsp kosher salt
- 1 tbsp. water
- 1/8 tsp pepper
- 1/4 tsp lemon juice
- 1/2 tsp lemon zest
- 1 tbsps. Chives, minced

Directions:

1. In a bowl that is save to microwave, add the cauliflower, mayo, garlic, water, and salt/pepper and mix until the cauliflower is well coated. Cook on high for 15-18 minutes, until the cauliflower is almost mushy.
2. Blend the mixture in a strong blender until completely smooth, adding a little more water if the mixture is too chunky. Season with the remaining ingredients and serve.

Nutrition: Net carbs: 3g, Protein: 2g, Fat: 18g, Calories: 178kcal.

52. Wilted Beet Greens with Goat Cheese and Pine Nuts

Preparation Time: 25 minutes
Cooking Time: 30 minutes
Servings: 3
Ingredients:

- 4 cups beet tops, washed and chopped roughly
- 1 tsp EVOO
- 1 tbsp. no sugar added balsamic vinegar
- 2 oz. crumbled dry goat cheese
- 2 tbsps. Toasted pine nuts

Directions:

1. Heat the oil in a large pan, then cook the beet greens on medium high heat until they release their moisture. Let it cook until almost tender. Season with salt and pepper and remove from heat.
2. Toss the greens in a mixture of balsamic vinegar and olive oil, then top with the nuts and cheese. Serve warm.

Nutrition: Net carbs: 3.5g, Protein: 10g, Fat: 18g, Calories: 215kcal.

53. Eggplant Parmesan

Preparation Time: 1 hour 20 minutes
Cooking Time: 30 minutes
Servings: 4
Ingredients:

- 1 large eggplant
- 1/2 tsp salt
- 1 large egg
- 1 tbsp. almond milk
- 1/2 cup almond flour
- 1/2 cup coconut flour
- 1 tsp Italian Seasoning
- 1 cup parmesan cheese

- cup coconut oil for frying

Directions:
1. Cut the eggplant into 1/4" rounds. Sprinkle them with salt on a cookies sheet and reserve for 45=60 minutes/
2. Set up a standard breading station: whisk the eggs in one bowl and season, place the parmesan cheese in another bowl, and mix the flours and Italian seasoning together in a separate bowl and season.
3. Pat the eggplant dry, then dip each slice in the egg, then the cheese, and finally the flour. Heat the frying oil in a heavy bottomed saucepan.
4. When the oil is hot, drop the eggplant slices in and fry until golden brown on both sides. Turn the eggplant once you see a ring of golden brown just on the bottom edge of the eggplant. Each side should cook 3-5 minutes.
5. Drain on paper towels and season with salt as needed. Serve warm.

Nutrition: Net carbs: 7.3g, Protein: 16.2g, Fat: 31.2g, Calories: 405kcal.

54. Celeriac Cauliflower Mash

Preparation Time: 20 minutes
Cooking Time: 30 minutes
Servings: 6
Ingredients:
- 1 head cauliflower
- 1 small celery root
- 1/4 cup butter
- 1 tbsp. chopped rosemary
- 1 tbsp. chopped thyme
- 1 cup cream cheese

Directions:
1. Peel the celery root and cut into small pieces. Cut the cauliflower into similar sized pieces and combine.
2. Toast the herbs in the butter in a large pan, until they become fragrant. Add the cauliflower and celery root and stir to combine. Season and cook at medium high until whatever moisture is in the vegetables releases itself, then cover and cook on low for 10-12 minutes.
3. Once the vegetables are soft, remove from the heat and place them in the blender. Puree until very smooth, then add the cream cheese and puree again. Season and serve.

Nutrition: Net carbs: 7.3g, Protein: 5.6g, Fat: 20.8g, Calories: 225kcal.

55. Cheddar Drop Biscuits

Preparation Time: 30 minutes
Cooking Time: 30 minutes
Servings: 8
Ingredients:
- 1/4 cup coconut oil
- 4 eggs
- 2 tsp apple cider vinegar
- 1 1/2 cup coarse almond meal
- 1/2 tsp baking powder, gluten free
- 1/2 tsp onion powder
- 1/4 tsp salt
- 3/4 cup cheddar cheese
- 2 tbsps. Chopped jalapenos

Directions:
1. Line a sheet tray with parchment paper, then preheat the oven to 400F
2. Mix the wet ingredients in a bowl until combined, then reserve. Mix the dry ingredients in a separate bowl until combined, then add them to the wet ingredients, stirring until incorporated. Fold in the cheddar cheese and jalapenos.
3. Drop the dough onto the parchment paper into eight roughly equal pieces, then shape as desired once they are on the tray.
4. Bake until golden brown, 12-15 minutes. Rotate the tray halfway through baking so browning is even.
5. Cool slightly and serve.

Nutrition: Net carbs: 6.9g, Protein: 3.2g, Fat: 22.1g, Calories: 260kcal.

56. Roasted Radish with Fresh Herbs

Preparation Time: 15 minutes
Cooking Time: 30 minutes
Servings: 4
Ingredients:
- 1 tbsp. coconut oil
- 1 bunch radishes
- 2 tbsps. Minced chives
- 1 tbsp. minced rosemary
- 1 tbsp. minced thyme

Directions:
1. Wash the radishes, then remove the tops and stems. Cut them into quarters and reserve.
2. Add the oil to a cast iron pan, then heat to medium. Add the radishes, then season with salt and pepper. Cook on medium heat for 6-8 minutes, until almost tender, then add the herbs and cook through.
3. The radishes can be served warm with meats or chilled with salads.

Nutrition: Net carbs: 1.8g, Protein: .9g, Fat: 13g, Calories: 133kcal.

57. Summer Bruschetta

Preparation Time: 15 min
Cooking Time: 30 minutes
Servings: 4
Ingredients:
- Basil leaves (chopped): 6
- Artichoke hearts (quartered): ½ cup
- Kalamata olives (halved): ¼ cup
- Capers: ¼ cup
- Roma tomatoes (diced): 4
- Balsamic vinegar: 3 tablespoon
- Avocado oil: 3 tablespoon
- Onion powder: ¾ teaspoon
- Sea salt: ¾ teaspoon
- Black pepper: ½ teaspoon

- Garlic (minced): 2 tablespoon

Directions:

1. Combine all the ingredients in the slow cooker and stir mix.
2. Cook for 3 hours on high, stirring the mix after every hour.

Nutrition: 152 Cal, 13g total fat, 7.5 g net carb., 1 g protein.

58.   Herbed Garlic Mushrooms

Preparation Time: 10 min
Cooking Time: 3-4 hours
Servings: 4
Ingredients:

- Cremini mushrooms: 24 oz.
- Garlic cloves (minced): 4
- Dried basil: ½ teaspoon
- Dried oregano: ½ teaspoon
- Dried thyme: ¼ teaspoon
- Bay leaves: 2
- Vegetable broth: 1 cup
- Half-and-half: ¼ cup
- Unsalted butter: 2 tablespoon
- Fresh parsley leaves (chopped): 2 tablespoon
- Kosher salt and black pepper: to taste

Directions:

1. Combine all the ingredients except the butter, half and half and fresh parsley in a slow cooker.
2. Cook covered for 3-4 hours on low.
3. 20 minutes prior to the completion of cook time, mix in the butter and half-and-half.
4. Garnish with parsley and serve.

Nutrition: 120 Cal, 8 g fat, 20 mg chol., 450 mg sodium, 7 g net carb., 2 g fiber, 6 g protein.

59.   Brussels Sprouts with Cashew Dip

Preparation Time: 20 min
Cooking Time: 15 min
Servings: 10
Ingredients:

- Extra-virgin olive oil: 2 tablespoons
- Brussels sprouts (ends trimmed): 1 lb.
- Salt: ½ teaspoon
- Pepper: ¼ teaspoon
- Dip:
- Silk Cashew milk (unsweetened): 1 cup
- Garlic clove (minced): 1
- Lemon juice: 3 tablespoon
- Cashew butter (unsweetened): 1 ½ cups
- Coarse sea salt: ½ teaspoon
- Black pepper: 2 teaspoon

Directions:

1. Toss together the sprouts, with salt, pepper and oil.
2. Roast in an oven preheated to 400 degrees Fahrenheit for 12-15 minutes and place aside.
3. For the cashew dip, combine all the dip ingredients in a blender and blend until smooth.
4. Serve the sprouts with the dip.

Nutrition: 221 Cal, 17 g total fat (3 g sat. fat), 0 mg chol., 241 mg sodium, 12.9 g carb., 1.3 g fiber, 7.4 g protein.

60.   Spaghetti Squash Mash

Preparation Time: 5 min
Cooking Time: 1 hour
Servings: 4
Ingredients:

- Spaghetti squash (halved, seeds removed) - 1
- Olive oil: 2 tablespoon
- Garlic powder: 1 teaspoon
- Dried rosemary: 1 teaspoon
- Dried parsley: 1 teaspoon
- Dried thyme: 1 teaspoon
- Sage: ½ teaspoon
- Salt: 1 teaspoon
- Cracked pepper: ½ teaspoon

Directions:

1. Put a little water in a baking pan and place the squash halves in it, cut side down.
2. Roast in an oven preheated to 350 degrees Fahrenheit for 45 minutes to an hour.
3. Remove, leave to cool and then scoop out all the flesh.
4. Place the squash in a bowl and mix in the rest of the ingredients.
5. Place in the oven and cook for 15 minutes more.

Nutrition: 91 Cal, 7 g total fat, 5.5 g net carb., 1.5 g fiber, 3 g protein.

61.   Avocado Hummus

Preparation Time: 10 min
Cooking Time: 30 minutes
Servings: 4
Ingredients:

- Zucchini (peeled, cubed) - 1
- Lemon (juice): ½
- Avocado (peeled, pitted, cubed) - 1
- Creamy roasted tahini (with salt): ¼ cup
- Olive oil: 1 tablespoon
- Garlic cloves (minced): 3
- Cumin: 1 teaspoon
- Sea salt: 1 teaspoon

Directions:

1. Combine all the ingredients in a food processor.
2. Process until smooth.
3. Refrigerate for 3-4 hours.

Nutrition: 80 Cal, 7.2 g total fat, 2.4 g net carb., 2 g protein.

62.   Squash & Zucchini

Preparation Time: 5 min
Cooking Time: 4-6 hours
Servings: 6
Ingredients:

- Zucchini (sliced and quartered): 2 cups
- Yellow squash (sliced and quartered): 2 cups
- Pepper: ¼ teaspoon
- Italian seasoning: 1 teaspoon
- Garlic powder: 1 teaspoon

- Sea salt: ½ teaspoon
- Butter (cubed): ¼ cup
- Parmesan cheese (grated): ¼ cup

Directions:
1. Combine all the ingredients in the slow cooker.
2. Cook covered for 4-6 hours on low.

Nutrition: 122 Cal, 9.9 g fat, 369 mg sodium, 5.4 g carb., 1.7 g fiber, 4.2 g protein.

63. **Roasted Broccoli**

Preparation Time: 5 min
Cooking Time: 15 min
Servings: 4
Ingredients:

- Broccoli (separated into florets) - 2
- Extra-virgin olive oil: ¼ cup
- Garlic cloves (minced): 2
- Lemon juice: 2 tablespoon
- Salt: ½ teaspoon

Directions:
1. Toss together all the ingredients and place in a baking dish.
2. Roast in an oven preheated to 450 degrees Fahrenheit for 12-15 minutes until crispy tender.

Nutrition: 179 Cal, 14.3 g total fat (8.3 g sat. fat) 10.9 g carb., 3.9 g fiber, 4.3 g protein.

64. **Avocado and Cauliflower Hummus**

Preparation Time: 20 minutes
Cooking Time: 20 minutes
Servings: 2
Ingredients:

- 1 medium cauliflower (stem removed and chopped)
- 1 large Hass avocado (peeled, pitted, and chopped)
- ¼ cup extra virgin olive oil
- garlic cloves
- ½ tbsp. lemon juice
- ½ tsp. onion powder
- Sea salt and ground black pepper to taste
- large carrots (peeled and cut into fries, or use store-bought raw carrot fries)
- Optional: ¼ cup fresh cilantro (chopped)

Directions:
1. Preheat the oven to 450°F/220°C, and line a baking tray with aluminum foil.
2. Put the chopped cauliflower on the baking tray and drizzle with 2 tablespoons of olive oil.
3. Roast the chopped cauliflower in the oven for 20-25 minutes, until lightly brown.
4. Remove the tray from the oven and allow the cauliflower to cool down.
5. Add all the ingredients—except the carrots and optional fresh cilantro—to a food processor or blender, and blend the ingredients into a smooth hummus.
6. Transfer the hummus to a medium-sized bowl, cover, and put it in the fridge for at least 30 minutes.

7. Take the hummus out of the fridge and, if desired, top it with the optional chopped cilantro and more salt and pepper to taste; serve with the carrot fries, and enjoy!
8. Alternatively, store it in the fridge in an airtight container, and consume within 2 days.

Nutrition: Calories: 416 kcal Net Carbs: 8.4 g. Fat: 40.3 g. Protein: 3.3 g. Fiber: 10.3 g. Sugar: 7.1 g.

65. **Peppers Rice**

Preparation Time: 10 minutes
Cooking Time: 25 minutes
Servings: 4
Ingredients:

- yellow bell pepper, chopped
- 1 red bell pepper, chopped
- green bell pepper, chopped
- scallions, chopped
- cups cauliflower rice
- cup vegetable stock
- 1 tablespoon olive oil
- teaspoon coriander, ground
- 1 teaspoon cumin, ground
- teaspoon basil, dried
- 1 teaspoon oregano, dried
- A pinch of salt and black pepper
- tablespoon chives, chopped

Directions:
1. Heat up a pan with the oil over medium heat, add the scallions and the peppers and sauté for 5 minutes.
2. Add the cauliflower rice and the other ingredients, toss, cook over medium heat for 20 minutes, divide between plates and serve as a side dish.

Nutrition: Calories 69 Fat 4.4 Fiber 1.3 Carbs 8.9 Protein 1.3

66. **Cauliflower and Chives Mash**

Preparation Time: 10 minutes
Cooking Time: 20 minutes
Servings: 4
Ingredients:

- pounds cauliflower florets
- cups water
- teaspoon thyme, dried
- 1 teaspoon cumin, dried
- cup coconut cream
- garlic cloves, minced
- A pinch of salt and black pepper

Directions:
1. Put the cauliflower florets in a pot, add the water and the other ingredients except the cream, bring to a simmer and cook over medium heat for 20 minutes.
2. Drain the cauliflower, add the cream, mash everything with a potato masher, whisk well, divide between plates and serve.

Nutrition: Calories 200 Fat 14.7 Fiber 7.2 Carbs 16.3 Protein 6.1

67. Baked Artichokes and Green Beans

Preparation Time: 10 minutes
Cooking Time: 40 minutes
Servings: 4
Ingredients:

- 1 pound green beans, trimmed and halved
- scallions, chopped
- tablespoons olive oil
- 1 cup canned artichoke hearts, drained and quartered
- garlic cloves, minced
- 1/3 cup tomato passata
- A pinch of salt and black pepper
- teaspoons mustard powder
- 1 teaspoon cumin, ground
- 1 teaspoon coriander, ground

Directions:

1. Heat up a pan with the oil over medium heat, add the scallions and the garlic and sauté for 5 minutes.
2. Add the green beans and the other ingredients, toss, introduce in the oven and bake at 390 degrees F for 35 minutes.
3. Divide the mix between plates and serve as a side dish.

Nutrition: Calories 132 Fat 7.8 Fiber 6.9 Carbs 14.8 Protein 4.4

68. Cumin Cauliflower Rice and Broccoli

Preparation Time: 10 minutes
Cooking Time: 25 minutes
Servings: 4
Ingredients:

- cups cauliflower rice
- 1 cup broccoli florets
- tablespoons olive oil
- scallions, chopped
- 1 teaspoon sweet paprika
- 1 teaspoon chili powder
- 1 cup vegetable stock
- 1 teaspoon red pepper flakes
- A pinch of salt and black pepper
- ¼ teaspoon cumin, ground

Directions:

1. Heat up a pan with the oil over medium heat, add the scallions, paprika and chili powder and sauté for 5 minutes.
2. Add the cauliflower rice and the other ingredients, toss, bring to a simmer, cook over medium heat for 20 minutes, divide between plates and serve.

Nutrition: Calories 81 Fat 7.9 Fiber 1.5 Carbs 4.1 Protein 1.1

69. Turmeric Cauliflower Rice and Tomatoes

Preparation Time: 10 minutes
Cooking Time: 25 minutes
Servings: 4
Ingredients:

- 2 tablespoons olive oil
- 2 cups cauliflower rice
- 2 scallions, chopped
- 2 garlic cloves, minced
- 1 cup cherry tomatoes, halved
- 1 teaspoon basil, dried
- 1 teaspoon oregano, dried
- A pinch of salt and black pepper
- ¼ teaspoon turmeric powder
- 1 cup vegetable stock
- A handful cilantro, chopped

Directions:

1. Heat up a pan with the oil over medium heat, add the scallions, garlic, basil, oregano and turmeric and sauté for 5 minutes.
2. Add the cauliflower rice, tomatoes and the remaining ingredients, toss, cook over medium heat for 20 minutes, divide between plates and serve as a side dish.

Nutrition: Calories 77 Fat 7.7 Fiber 1 Carbs 3.7 Protein 0.7

70. Flavored Tomato and Okra Mix

Preparation Time: 10 minutes
Cooking Time: 30 minutes
Servings: 6
Ingredients:

- 1 cup scallions, chopped
- 1-pound cherry tomatoes, halved
- cups okra, sliced
- tablespoons avocado oil
- garlic cloves, chopped
- teaspoons oregano, dried
- A pinch of salt and black pepper
- teaspoons cumin, ground
- 1 cup veggie stock
- tablespoons tomato passata

Directions:

1. Heat up a pan with the oil over medium heat, add the scallions and the garlic and sauté for 5 minutes.
2. Add the tomatoes, the okra and the other ingredients, toss, cook over medium heat for 25 minutes, divide between plates and serve as a side dish.

Nutrition: Calories 84 Fat 2.1 Fiber 5.4 Carbs 14.8 Protein 4

71. Orange Scallions and Brussels Sprouts

Preparation Time: 10 minutes
Cooking Time: 25 minutes
Servings: 4
Ingredients:

- pound Brussels sprouts, trimmed and halved
- 1 cup scallions, chopped
- Zest of 1 lime, grated
- tablespoon olive oil

- ¼ cup orange juice
- tablespoons stevia
- A pinch of salt and black pepper

Directions:
1. Heat up a pan with the oil over medium heat, add the scallions and sauté for 5 minutes.
2. Add the sprouts and the other ingredients, toss, cook over medium heat for 20 minutes more, divide the mix between plates and serve.

Nutrition: Calories 193 Fat 4 Fiber 1 Carbs 8 Protein 10

72. Roasted Artichokes and Sauce

Preparation Time: 10 minutes
Cooking Time: 30 minutes
Servings: 4
Ingredients:

- big artichokes, trimmed and halved
- tablespoons avocado oil
- Juice of 1 lime
- teaspoon turmeric powder
- 1 cup coconut cream
- A pinch of salt and black pepper
- ½ teaspoon onion powder
- ¼ teaspoon sweet paprika
- teaspoon cumin, ground

Directions:
1. In a roasting pan, combine the artichokes with the oil, the lime juice and the other ingredients, toss and bake at 390 degrees F for 30 minutes.
2. Divide the artichokes and sauce between plates and serve.

Nutrition: Calories 190 Fat 6 Fiber 8 Carbs 10 Protein 9

73. Zucchini Risotto

Preparation Time: 10 minutes
Cooking Time: 30 minutes
Servings: 4
Ingredients:

- ½ cup shallots, chopped
- tablespoons olive oil
- garlic cloves, minced
- cups cauliflower rice
- cup zucchinis, cubed
- cups veggie stock
- ½ cup white mushrooms, chopped
- ½ teaspoon coriander, ground
- A pinch of salt and black pepper
- ¼ teaspoon oregano, dried
- tablespoons parsley, chopped

Directions:
1. Heat up a pan with the oil over medium heat, add the shallots, garlic, mushrooms, coriander and oregano, stir and sauté for 10 minutes.
2. Add the cauliflower rice and the other ingredients, toss, cook for 20 minutes more, divide between plates and serve.

Nutrition: Calories 231 fat 5 fiber 3 carbs 9 protein 12

74. Cabbage and Rice

Preparation Time: 10 minutes
Cooking Time: 30 minutes
Servings: 4
Ingredients:

- cup green cabbage, shredded
- 1 cup cauliflower rice
- tablespoons olive oil
- tablespoons tomato passata
- spring onions, chopped
- teaspoons balsamic vinegar
- A pinch of salt and black pepper
- teaspoons fennel seeds, crushed
- teaspoon coriander, ground

Directions:
1. Heat up a pan with the oil over medium heat, add the spring onions, fennel and coriander, stir and cook for 5 minutes.
2. Add the cabbage, cauliflower rice and the other ingredients, toss, cook over medium heat for 25 minutes more, divide between plates and serve.

Nutrition: Calories 200 fat 4 fiber 1 carbs 8 protein 5

75. Tomato Risotto

Preparation Time: 10 minutes
Cooking Time: 30 minutes
Servings: 4
Ingredients:

- 1 cup shallots, chopped
- cups cauliflower rice
- tablespoons olive oil
- cups veggie stock
- 1 cup tomatoes, crushed
- ¼ cup cilantro, chopped
- ½ teaspoon chili powder
- 1 teaspoon cumin, ground
- 1 teaspoon coriander, ground

Directions:
1. Heat up a pan with the oil over medium heat, add the shallots and sauté for 5 minutes.
2. Add the cauliflower rice, tomatoes and the other ingredients, toss, cook over medium heat for 25 minutes more, divide between plates and serve.

Nutrition: Calories 200 Fat 4 Fiber 3 Carbs 6 Protein 8

76. Herbed Risotto

Preparation Time: 10 minutes
Cooking Time: 25 minutes
Servings: 4
Ingredients:

- cups cauliflower rice
- scallions, chopped
- tablespoons avocado oil
- cups veggie stock
- Juice of 1 lime
- 1 tablespoon parsley, chopped
- 1 tablespoon cilantro, chopped
- 1 tablespoon basil, chopped

- 1 tablespoon oregano, chopped
- 1 teaspoon sweet paprika
- A pinch of salt and black pepper

Directions:
1. Heat up a pan with the oil over medium heat, add the scallions and sauté for 5 minutes.
2. Add the cauliflower rice, the stock and the other ingredients, toss, cook over medium heat for 20 minutes, divide between plates and serve as a side dish.

Nutrition: Calories 182 fat 4 fiber 2 carbs 8 protein 10

77. Radish and Broccoli

Preparation Time: 10 minutes
Cooking Time: 30 minutes
Servings: 4
Ingredients:

- 1-pound broccoli florets
- 2 tablespoons olive oil
- scallions, chopped
- ½ pound radishes, halved
- garlic cloves, minced
- teaspoons cumin, ground
- tablespoons tomato passata
- ½ cup veggie stock
- A pinch of salt and black pepper

Directions:
1. Heat up a pan with the oil over medium heat, add the scallions and sauté for 5 minutes.
2. Add the broccoli, radishes and the other ingredients, toss, cook over medium heat for 25 minutes more, divide between plates and serve.

Nutrition: Calories 261 fat 5 fiber 4 carbs 9 protein 12

78. Mushrooms and Radishes Mix

Preparation Time: 10 minutes
Cooking Time: 25 minutes
Servings: 4
Ingredients:

- 1 pound white mushrooms, halved
- ½ pound radishes, halved
- scallions, chopped
- garlic cloves, minced
- tablespoons olive oil
- ½ cup veggie stock
- tablespoons parsley, chopped
- 1 teaspoon coriander, ground
- 1 teaspoon rosemary, dried
- A pinch of salt and black pepper

Directions:
1. Heat up a pan with the oil over medium heat, add the scallions, garlic, coriander and rosemary, stir and cook for 5 minutes.
2. Add the mushrooms, radishes and the other ingredients, toss, cook over medium heat for 20 minutes, divide between plates and serve as a side dish.

Nutrition: Calories 182 Fat 4 Fiber 2 Carbs 6 Protein 8

79. Summertime Vegetable Chicken Wraps

Preparation Time: 15 minutes
Cooking Time: 0 min
Serving: 4
Ingredients:

- 2 cups cooked chicken, chopped
- ½ English cucumbers, diced
- ½ red bell pepper, diced
- ½ cup carrot, shredded
- 1 scallion, white and green parts, chopped
- ¼ cup plain Greek yogurt
- 1 tablespoon freshly squeezed lemon juice
- ½ teaspoon fresh thyme, chopped
- Pinch of salt
- Pinch of ground black pepper
- 4 multigrain tortillas

Directions:
1. Take a medium bowl and mix in chicken, red bell pepper, cucumber, carrot, yogurt, scallion, lemon juice, thyme, sea salt and pepper.
2. Mix well.
3. Spoon one quarter of chicken mix into the middle of the tortilla and fold the opposite ends of the tortilla over the filling.
4. Roll the tortilla from the side to create a snug pocket.
5. Repeat with the remaining ingredients and serve.
6. Enjoy!

Nutrition: Calories: 278 Fat: 4g Carbohydrates: 28g Protein: 27g

80. Premium Roasted Baby Potatoes

Preparation Time: 10 minutes
Cook Time: 35 minutes
Serving: 4
Ingredients:

- 2 pounds' new yellow potatoes, scrubbed and cut into wedges
- 2 tablespoons extra virgin olive oil
- 2 teaspoons fresh rosemary, chopped
- 1 teaspoon garlic powder
- 1 teaspoon sweet paprika
- ½ teaspoon sea salt
- ½ teaspoon freshly ground black pepper

Directions:
1. Pre-heat your oven to 400 degrees Fahrenheit.
2. Line baking sheet with aluminum foil and set it aside.
3. Take a large bowl and add potatoes, olive oil, garlic, rosemary, paprika, sea salt and pepper.
4. Spread potatoes in single layer on baking sheet and bake for 35 minutes.
5. Serve and enjoy!

Nutrition: Calories: 225 Fat: 7g Carbohydrates: 37g Protein: 5g

81. Tomato and Cherry Linguine

Preparation Time: 10 minutes
Cooking Time: 15 minutes
Serving: 4
Ingredients:

- 2 pounds' cherry tomatoes
- 3 tablespoons extra virgin olive oil
- 2 tablespoons balsamic vinegar
- 2 teaspoons garlic, minced
- Pinch of fresh ground black pepper
- ¾ pound whole-wheat linguine pasta
- 1 tablespoon fresh oregano, chopped
- ¼ cup feta cheese, crumbled

Directions:

1. Pre-heat your oven to 350 degrees Fahrenheit.
2. Line baking sheet with parchment paper and keep aside.
3. Take a large bowl and add cherry tomatoes, 2 tablespoons olive oil, balsamic vinegar, garlic, pepper and toss.
4. Spread tomatoes evenly on baking sheet and roast for 15 minutes.
5. While the tomatoes are roasting, cook the pasta according to the package instructions and drain the paste into a large bowl.
6. Toss pasta with 1 tablespoon olive oil.
7. Add roasted tomatoes (with juice) and toss.
8. Serve with topping of oregano and feta cheese.
9. Enjoy!

Nutrition: Calories: 397 Fat: 15g Carbohydrates: 55g Protein: 13g

82. Mediterranean Zucchini Mushroom Pasta

Preparation Time: 10 minutes
Cooking Time: 10 minutes
Servings: 4
Ingredients:

- ½ pound pasta
- 2 tablespoons olive oil
- 6 garlic cloves, crushed
- 1 teaspoon red chili
- 2 spring onions, sliced
- 3 teaspoons rosemary, chopped
- 1 large zucchini, cut in half lengthwise and sliced
- 5 large portabella mushrooms
- 1 can tomatoes
- 4 tablespoons Parmesan cheese
- Fresh ground black pepper

Directions:

1. Cook the pasta in boiling water until Al Dente.
2. Take a large-sized frying pan and place it over medium heat.
3. Add oil and allow the oil to heat up.
4. Add garlic, onion and chili and sauté for a few minutes until golden.
5. Add zucchini, rosemary and mushroom and sauté for a few minutes.

6. Increase the heat to medium-high and add tinned tomatoes to the sauce until thick.
7. Drain your boiled pasta and transfer to serving platter.
8. Pour the tomato mix on top and mix using tongs.
9. Garnish with Parmesan and freshly ground black pepper.
10. Enjoy!

Nutrition: Calories: 361 Fat: 12g Carbohydrates: 47g Protein: 14g

83. Lemon and Garlic Fettucine

Preparation Time: 5 minutes
Cooking Time: 15 minutes
Servings: 5
Ingredients:

- 8 ounces of whole wheat fettuccine
- 4 tablespoons of extra virgin olive oil
- 4 cloves of minced garlic
- 1 cup of fresh breadcrumbs
- ¼ cup of lemon juice
- 1 teaspoon of freshly ground pepper
- ½ teaspoon of salt
- 2 cans of 4 ounce boneless and skinless sardines (dipped in tomato sauce)
- ½ cup of chopped up fresh parsley
- ¼ cup of finely shredded Parmesan cheese

Directions:

1. Take a large-sized pot and bring water to a boil.
2. Cook pasta for 10 minutes until Al Dente.
3. Take a small-sized skillet and place it over medium heat.
4. Add 2 tablespoons of oil and allow it to heat up.
5. Add garlic and cook for 20 seconds.
6. Transfer the garlic to a medium-sized bowl
7. Add breadcrumbs to the hot skillet and cook for 5-6 minutes until golden
8. Whisk in lemon juice, pepper and salt into the garlic bowl
9. Add pasta to the bowl (with garlic) and sardines, parsley and Parmesan
10. Stir well and sprinkle bread crumbs
11. Enjoy!

Nutrition: Calories: 480 Fat: 21g Carbohydrates: 53g Protein: 23g

84. Roasted Broccoli with Parmesan

Preparation Time: 10 minutes
Cooking Time: 10 minutes
Servings: 4
Ingredients:

- 2 head broccoli, cut into florets
- 2 tablespoons extra-virgin olive oil
- 2 teaspoons garlic, minced
- Zest of 1 lemon
- Pinch of salt
- ½ cup Parmesan cheese, grated

Directions:

1. Pre-heat your oven to 400 degrees Fahrenheit.
2. Lightly grease the baking sheet with olive oil and keep it aside.
3. Take a large bowl and add broccoli with 2 tablespoons olive oil, lemon zest, garlic, lemon juice and salt.
4. Spread mix on the baking sheet in single layer and sprinkle with Parmesan cheese.
5. Bake for 10 minutes until tender.
6. Transfer broccoli to serving the dish.
7. Serve and enjoy!

Nutrition: Calories: 154 Fat: 11g Carbohydrates: 10g Protein: 9g

85.   Spinach and Feta Bread

Preparation Time: 10 minutes
Cooking Time: 12 minute
Serving: 6
Ingredients:

- 6 ounces of sun dried tomato pesto
- 6 pieces of 6-inch whole wheat pita bread
- 2 chopped up Roma plum tomatoes
- 1 bunch of rinsed and chopped spinach
- 4 sliced fresh mushrooms
- ½ cup of crumbled feta cheese
- 2 tablespoons of grated Parmesan cheese
- 3 tablespoons of olive oil
- Ground black pepper as needed

Directions:

1. Pre-heat your oven to a temperature of 350 degrees Fahrenheit.
2. Spread your tomato pesto onto one side of your pita bread and place on your baking sheet (with the pesto side up).
3. Top up the pitas with spinach, tomatoes, feta cheese, mushrooms and Parmesan cheese.
4. Drizzle with some olive oil and season nicely with pepper.
5. Bake in your oven for about 12 minutes until the breads are crispy.
6. Cut up the pita into quarters and serve!

Nutrition: Calories: 350 Fat: 17g Carbohydrates: 41g Protein:11g

86.   Quick Zucchini Bowl

Preparation Time: 10 minutes
Cooking Time: 10 minutes
Servings: 4
Ingredients:

- ½ pound of pasta
- 2 tablespoons of olive oil
- 6 crushed garlic cloves
- 1 teaspoon of red chili
- 2 finely sliced spring onions
- 3 teaspoons of chopped rosemary
- 1 large zucchini cut up in half, lengthways and sliced
- 5 large portabella mushrooms
- 1 can of tomatoes

- 4 tablespoons of Parmesan cheese
- Fresh ground black pepper

Directions:

1. Cook the pasta in boiling water until Al Dente.
2. Take a large-sized frying pan and place over medium heat.
3. Add oil and allow the oil to heat up.
4. Add garlic, onion and chili and sauté for a few minutes until golden.
5. Add zucchini, rosemary and mushroom and sauté for a few minutes.
6. Increase the heat to medium-high and add tinned tomatoes to the sauce until thick.
7. Drain your boiled pasta and transfer to a serving platter.
8. Pour the tomato mix on top and mix using tongs.
9. Garnish with Parmesan cheese and freshly ground black pepper.
10. Enjoy!

Nutrition: Calories: 361 Fat: 12g Carbohydrates: 47g Protein: 14g

87.   Healthy Basil Platter

Preparation Time: 25 minutes
Cooking Time: 15 minutes
Servings: 4
Ingredients:

- 2 pieces of red pepper seeded and cut up into chunks
- 2 pieces of red onion cut up into wedges
- 2 mild red chilies, diced and seeded
- 3 coarsely chopped garlic cloves
- 1 teaspoon of golden caster sugar
- 2 tablespoons of olive oil (plus additional for serving)
- 2 pound of small ripe tomatoes quartered up
- 12 ounces of dried pasta
- Just a handful of basil leaves
- 2 tablespoons of grated Parmesan

Directions:

1. Pre-heat the oven to 392 degrees Fahrenheit.
2. Take a large-sized roasting tin and scatter pepper, red onion, garlic and chilies.
3. Sprinkle sugar on top.
4. Drizzle olive oil and season with pepper and salt.
5. Roast the veggies in your oven for 15 minutes.
6. Take a large-sized pan and cook the pasta in boiling, salted water until Al Dente.
7. Drain them.
8. Remove the veggies from the oven and tip in the pasta into the veggies.
9. Toss well and tear basil leaves on top.
10. Sprinkle Parmesan and enjoy!

Nutrition: Calories: 452 Fat: 8g Carbohydrates: 88g Protein:14g

88.   Herbed Up Bruschetta

Preparation Time: 12 minutes
Cooking Time: 0 minute
Servings: 12

Ingredients:

- 16 thin slices of toasted French bread
- 2 cups of quartered cherry tomatoes
- 1 finely chopped medium-sized white onion
- Salt as needed
- Ground black pepper as needed
- Fresh sweet basil
- For dressing
- ¼ cup of olive oil
- 2 tablespoons of balsamic vinegar
- 1 tablespoon of lemon juice
- 1 tablespoon of Dijon mustard
- 2 tablespoons of minced fresh herbs
- 1 minced clove of garlic

Directions:

1. Whisk together your olive oil, lemon juice, balsamic vinegar, Dijon mustard, garlic and mixed herbs in a medium-sized bowl.
2. Add the onion and cherry tomatoes.
3. Toss finely to coat it.
4. Season with some pepper and salt.
5. Top each of your bread toast with the previously made tomato mix.
6. Drizzle with some more dressing if you like.
7. Garnish it with fresh basil.
8. Serve.

Nutrition: Calories: 118 Fat: 4g Carbohydrates: 18g Protein: 4g

89. **Homemade Almond Biscotti**

Preparation Time: 10 minutes
Cooking Time: 35 minutes
Servings: 30
Ingredients:

- 2/3 cups of soft unsalted butter
- ¾ cup and 2 tablespoons of granulated sugar
- 1 teaspoon of crushed anise seed
- 2 whole sized eggs
- 2 tablespoons of amaretto liqueur
- 1 teaspoon of vanilla extract
- 2 ¼ cup of all-purpose flour
- 1 teaspoon of baking powder
- 1 teaspoon of baking soda
- ½ teaspoon of salt
- ¾ cup of chopped up roasted almonds

Directions:

1. Pre-heat your oven to a temperature of 325 degrees Fahrenheit.
2. Line a cookie sheet with parchment paper.
3. Take an electric mixer and cream your butter.
4. Then, slowly add the sugar and keep mixing until light and fluffy.
5. Add the aniseed.
6. Add the eggs one at a time, making sure to mix after every addition.
7. Stir in your amaretto liqueur alongside the vanilla extract.

8. Slowly add the flour, baking soda and baking powder.
9. Fold in the chopped up almonds.
10. Divide the dough into 2 halves with floured dusted hands and form each of the dough into a rough 12 x 2 and a ½ inch log.
11. Bake your logs for 25 minutes until a fine golden brown texture appears.
12. Cool them on a wire rack.
13. Slice your logs diagonally into ½ inch wide pieces using a serrated knife.
14. Place them in your cookie sheet to make one single layer.
15. Return them to your oven and bake for another 7 minutes until the edges are browned.
16. Serve.

Nutrition: Calories: 111 Fat: 6g Carbohydrates: 13g Protein: 2g

90. **Lemon Garlic Green Beans**

Preparation Time: 5 minutes
Cooking Time: 10 minutes
Servings: 6
Ingredients:

- 1 ½ pounds green beans, trimmed
- 2 tablespoons olive oil
- 1-tablespoon fresh lemon juice
- Two cloves minced garlic
- Salt and pepper

Directions:

1. Fill a large bowl with ice water and set aside.
2. Bring a pot of salted water to boil then add the green beans.
3. Cook for 3 minutes then drain and immediately place in the ice water.
4. Cool the beans completely then drain them well.
5. Heat the oil in a large skillet over medium-high heat.
6. Add the green beans, tossing to coat, then add the lemon juice, garlic, salt, and pepper.
7. Sauté for 3 minutes until the beans are tender-crisp then serve hot.

Nutrition: Calories 75 Total Fat 4.8g Saturated Fat 0.7g Total Carbs 8.5g Net Carbs 4.6g Protein 2.1g Sugar 1.7g Fiber 3.9g Sodium 7mg

91. **Brown Rice & Lentil Salad**

Preparation Time: 10 minutes
Cooking Time: 10 minutes
Servings: 4
Ingredients:

- 1-cup water
- ½ cup instant brown rice
- 2 tablespoons olive oil
- 2 tablespoons red wine vinegar
- 1-tablespoon Dijon mustard
- 1 tablespoon minced onion
- ½-teaspoon paprika
- Salt and pepper
- 1 (15-ounce) can brown lentils, rinsed and drained

- 1 medium carrot, shredded
- 2 tablespoons fresh chopped parsley

Directions:
1. Stir together the water and instant brown rice in a medium saucepan.
2. Bring to a boil then simmer for 10 minutes, covered.
3. Remove from heat and set aside while you prepare the salad.
4. Whisk together the olive oil, vinegar, Dijon mustard, onion, paprika, salt, and pepper in a medium bowl.
5. Toss in the cooked rice, lentils, carrots, and parsley.
6. Adjust seasoning to taste then stir well and serve warm.

Nutrition: Calories 1455 Total Fat 4.8g Saturated Fat 0.7g Total Carbs 8.5g Net Carbs 4.6g Protein 2.1g Sugar 1.7g Fiber 3.9g Sodium 75mg

92. **Mashed Butternut Squash**

Preparation Time: 5 minutes
Cooking Time: 25 minutes
Servings: 6
Ingredients:
- 3 pounds' whole butternut squash (about 2 medium)
- 2 tablespoons olive oil
- Salt and pepper

Directions:
1. Preheat the oven to 400°F and line a baking sheet with parchment.
2. Cut the squash in half and remove the seeds.
3. Cut the squash into cubes and toss with oil then spread on the baking sheet.
4. Roast for 25 minutes until tender then place in a food processor.
5. Blend smooth then season with salt and pepper to taste.

Nutrition: Calories 90 Total Fat 4.8g Saturated Fat 0.7g Total Carbs 8.5g Net Carbs 4.6g Protein 2.1g Sugar 1.7g Fiber 3.9g Sodium 4mg

93. **Cilantro Lime Quinoa**

Preparation Time: 5 minutes
Cooking Time: 25 minutes
Servings: 6
Ingredients:
- 1 cup uncooked quinoa
- 1-tablespoon olive oil
- 1 medium yellow onion, diced
- 2 cloves minced garlic
- 1 (4-ounce) can diced green chills, drained
- 1 ½ cups fat-free chicken broth
- ¾-cup fresh chopped cilantro
- ½ cup sliced green onion
- 2 tablespoons lime juice
- Salt and pepper

Directions:
1. Rinse the quinoa thoroughly in cool water using a fine mesh sieve.

2. Heat the oil in a large saucepan over medium heat.
3. Add the onion and sauté for 2 minutes then stir in the chili and garlic.
4. Cook for 1 minute then stir in the quinoa and chicken broth.
5. Bring to a boil then reduce heat and simmer, covered, until the quinoa absorbs the liquid: about 20 to 25 minutes.
6. Remove from heat then stir in the cilantro, green onions, and limejuice.
7. Season with salt and pepper to taste and serve hot.

Nutrition: Calories 150 Total Fat 4.8g Saturated Fat 0.7g Total Carbs 8.5g Net Carbs 4.6g Protein 2.1g Sugar 1.7g Fiber 3.9g Sodium 179mg

94. **Oven-Roasted Veggies**

Preparation Time: 5 minutes
Cooking Time: 25 minutes
Servings: 6
Ingredients:
- 1-pound cauliflower florets
- ½-pound broccoli florets
- 1 large yellow onion, cut into chunks
- 1 large red pepper, cored and chopped
- 2 medium carrots, peeled and sliced
- 2 tablespoons olive oil
- 2 tablespoons apple cider vinegar
- Salt and pepper

Directions:
1. Preheat the oven to 425°F and line a large rimmed baking sheet with parchment.
2. Spread the veggies on the baking sheet and drizzle with oil and vinegar.
3. Toss well and season with salt and pepper.
4. Spread the veggies in a single layer then roast for 20 to 25 minutes, stirring every 10 minutes, until tender.
5. Adjust seasoning to taste and serve hot.

Nutrition: Calories 100 Total Fat 4.8g Saturated Fat 0.7g Total Carbs 8.5g Net Carbs 4.6g Protein 2.1g Sugar 1.7g Fiber 3.9g Sodium 7mg

95. **Vegetable Rice Pilaf**

Preparation Time: 5 minutes
Cooking Time: 25 minutes
Servings: 6
Ingredients:
- 1-tablespoon olive oil
- ½ medium yellow onion, diced
- 1 cup uncooked long-grain brown rice
- 2 cloves minced garlic
- ½ teaspoon dried basil
- Salt and pepper
- 2 cups fat-free chicken broth
- 1 cup frozen mixed veggies

Directions:
1. Heat the oil in a large skillet over medium heat.
2. Add the onion and sauté for 3 minutes until translucent.
3. Stir in the rice and cook until lightly toasted.

4. Add the garlic, basil, salt, and pepper then stir to combine.
5. Stir in the chicken broth then bring to a boil.
6. Reduce heat and simmer, covered, for 10 minutes.
7. Stir in the frozen veggies then cover and cook for another 10 minutes until heated through. Serve hot.

Nutrition: Calories 75 Total Fat 4.8g Saturated Fat 0.7g Total Carbs 8.5g Net Carbs 4.6g Protein 2.1g Sugar 1.7g Fiber 3.9g Sodium 7mg

96. Curry Roasted Cauliflower Florets

Preparation Time: 5 minutes
Cooking Time: 25 minutes
Servings: 6
Ingredients:

- 8 cups cauliflower florets
- 2 tablespoons olive oil
- 1-teaspoon curry powder
- ½-teaspoon garlic powder
- Salt and pepper

Directions:

1. Preheat the oven to 425°F and line with foil.
2. Toss the cauliflower with the olive oil and spread on the baking sheet.
3. Sprinkle with curry powder, garlic powder, salt, and pepper.
4. Roast for 25 minutes or until just tender. Serve hot.

Nutrition: Calories 75 Total Fat 4.8g Saturated Fat 0.7g Total Carbs 8.5g Net Carbs 4.6g Protein 2.1g Sugar 1.7g Fiber 3.9g Sodium 40mg

97. Mushroom Barley Risotto

Preparation Time: 5 minutes
Cooking Time: 25 minutes
Servings: 8
Ingredients:

- 4 cups fat-free beef broth
- 2 tablespoons olive oil
- 1 small onion, diced well
- 2 cloves minced garlic
- 8 ounces thinly sliced mushrooms
- ¼ tsp. dried thyme

- Salt and pepper
- 1 cup pearled barley
- ½ cup dry white wine

Directions:

1. Heat the beef broth in a medium saucepan and keep it warm.
2. Heat the oil in a large, deep skillet over medium heat.
3. Add the onions, garlic, and sauté for 2 minutes then stir in the mushrooms and thyme.
4. Season with salt, pepper, and sauté for 2 minutes more.
5. Add the barley and sauté for 1 minute then pour in the wine.
6. Ladle about ½ cup of beef broth into the skillet and stir well to combine.
7. Cook until most of the broth has been absorbed then add another ladle.
8. Repeat until you have used all of the broth and the barley is cooked to al dente.
9. Adjust seasoning to taste with salt and pepper and serve hot.

Nutrition: Calories 1555 Total Fat 4.8g Saturated Fat 0.7g Total Carbs 8.5g Net Carbs 4.6g Protein 2.1g Sugar 1.7g Fiber 3.9g Sodium 445mg

98. Peaches and Cream Oatmeal Smoothie

Preparation time: 5 minutes
Cooking Time: 0 minutes
Servings: 1
Ingredients:

- Frozen peach slices: 1 cup
- Greek yogurt: 1 cup
- Oatmeal: ¼ cup
- Vanilla extract: ¼ tsp.
- Almond milk: 1 cup

Directions:

1. Combine everything in a blender and blend until smooth.

Nutrition: Calories: 331 Fat: 4 Carb: 46g Protein: 29g

SALAD RECIPES

99. Tuna salad

Preparation Time: 10 minutes
Cooking time: none
Servings: 3
Ingredients:

- 1 can tuna (6 oz)
- ⅓ cup fresh cucumber, chopped
- ⅓ cup fresh tomato, chopped
- ⅓ cup avocado, chopped
- ⅓ cup celery, chopped
- 2 garlic cloves, minced
- 4 tsp olive oil
- 2 tbsp lime juice
- Pinch of black pepper

Directions:

1. Prepare the dressing by combining olive oil, lime juice, minced garlic and black pepper.
2. Mix the salad ingredients in a salad bowl and drizzle with the dressing.

Nutrition: Carbohydrates: 4.8 g Protein: 14.3 g Total sugars: 1.1 g Calories: 212 g

100. Roasted Portobello Salad

Preparation Time: 10 minutes
Cooking time: none
Servings: 4
Ingredients:

- 1½ lb Portobello mushrooms, stems trimmed
- 3 heads Belgian endive, sliced
- 1 small red onion, sliced
- 4 oz blue cheese
- 8 oz mixed salad greens
- Dressing:
- 3 tbsp red wine vinegar
- 1 tbsp Dijon mustard
- ⅔ cup olive oil
- Salt and pepper to taste

Directions:

1. Preheat the oven to 450°F.
2. Prepare the dressing by whisking together vinegar, mustard, salt and pepper. Slowly add olive oil while whisking.
3. Cut the mushrooms and arrange them on a baking sheet, stem-side up. Coat the mushrooms with some dressing and bake for 15 minutes.
4. In a salad bowl toss the salad greens with onion, endive and cheese. Sprinkle with the dressing.
5. Add mushrooms to the salad bowl.

Nutrition: Carbohydrates: 22.3 g Protein: 14.9 g Total sugars: 2.1 g Calories: 501

101. Shredded chicken salad

Preparation Time: 5 minutes
Cooking time: 10 minutes
Servings: 6
Ingredients:

- 2 chicken breasts, boneless, skinless
- 1 head iceberg lettuce, cut into strips
- 2 bell peppers, cut into strips
- 1 fresh cucumber, quartered, sliced
- 3 scallions, sliced
- 2 tbsp chopped peanuts
- 1 tbsp peanut vinaigrette
- Salt to taste
- 1 cup water

Directions:

1. In a skillet simmer one cup of salted water.
2. Add the chicken breasts, cover and cook on low for 5 minutes. Remove the cover. Then remove the chicken from the skillet and shred with a fork.
3. In a salad bowl mix the vegetables with the cooled chicken, season with salt and sprinkle with peanut vinaigrette and chopped peanuts.

Nutrition: Carbohydrates: 9 g Protein: 11.6 g Total sugars: 4.2 g Calories: 117

102. Broccoli Salad

Preparation Time: 10 minutes
Cooking time: none
Servings: 6
Ingredients:

- 1 medium head broccoli, raw, florets only
- ½ cup red onion, chopped
- 12 oz turkey bacon, chopped, fried until crisp
- ½ cup cherry tomatoes, halved
- ¼ cup sunflower kernels
- ¾ cup raisins
- ¾ cup mayonnaise
- 2 tbsp white vinegar

Directions:

1. In a salad bowl combine the broccoli, tomatoes and onion.
2. Mix mayo with vinegar and sprinkle over the broccoli.
3. Add the sunflower kernels, raisins and bacon and toss well.

Nutrition: Carbohydrates: 17.3 g Protein: 11 g Total sugars: 10 g Calories: 220

103. Cherry Tomato Salad

Preparation Time: 10 minutes
Cooking time: none
Servings: 6
Ingredients:

- 40 cherry tomatoes, halved
- 1 cup mozzarella balls, halved
- 1 cup green olives, sliced
- 1 can (6 oz) black olives, sliced
- 2 green onions, chopped
- 3 oz roasted pine nuts
- Dressing:
- ½ cup olive oil

- 2 tbsp red wine vinegar
- 1 tsp dried oregano
- Salt and pepper to taste

Directions:

1. In a salad bowl, combine the tomatoes, olives and onions.
2. Prepare the dressing by combining olive oil with red wine vinegar, dried oregano, salt and pepper.
3. Sprinkle with the dressing and add the nuts.
4. Let marinate in the fridge for 1 hour.

Nutrition: Carbohydrates: 10.7 g Protein: 2.4 g Total sugars: 3.6 g

104. Ground turkey salad

Preparation Time: 10 minutes
Cooking time: 35 minutes
Servings: 6
Ingredients:

- 1 lb lean ground turkey
- ½ inch ginger, minced
- 2 garlic cloves, minced
- 1 onion, chopped
- 1 tbsp olive oil
- 1 bag lettuce leaves (for serving)
- ¼ cup fresh cilantro, chopped
- 2 tsp coriander powder
- 1 tsp red chili powder
- 1 tsp turmeric powder
- Salt to taste
- 4 cups water
- Dressing:
- 2 tbsp fat free yogurt
- 1 tbsp sour cream, non-fat
- 1 tbsp low fat mayonnaise
- 1 lemon, juiced
- 1 tsp red chili flakes
- Salt and pepper to taste

Directions:

1. In a skillet sauté the garlic and ginger in olive oil for 1 minute. Add onion and season with salt. Cook for 10 minutes over medium heat.
2. Add the ground turkey and sauté for 3 more minutes. Add the spices (turmeric, red chili powder and coriander powder).
3. Add 4 cups water and cook for 30 minutes, covered.
4. Prepare the dressing by combining yogurt, sour cream, mayo, lemon juice, chili flakes, salt and pepper.
5. To serve arrange the salad leaves on serving plates and place the cooked ground turkey on them. Top with dressing.

Nutrition: Carbohydrates: 9.1 g Protein: 17.8 g Total sugars: 2.5 g Calories: 176

105. Asian Cucumber Salad

Preparation Time: 10 minutes
Cooking time: none
Servings: 6

Ingredients:

- 1 lb cucumbers, sliced
- 2 scallions, sliced
- 2 tbsp sliced pickled ginger, chopped
- ¼ cup cilantro
- ½ red jalapeño, chopped
- 3 tbsp rice wine vinegar
- 1 tbsp sesame oil
- 1 tbsp sesame seeds

Directions:

1. In a salad bowl combine all ingredients and toss together.

Nutrition: Carbohydrates: 5.7 g Protein: 1 g Total sugars: 3.1 g Calories: 52

106. Cauliflower Tofu Salad

Preparation time: 10 minutes
Cooking time: 15 minutes
Servings: 4
Ingredients:

- 2 cups cauliflower florets, blended
- 1 fresh cucumber, diced
- ½ cup green olives, diced
- ⅓ cup red onion, diced
- 2 tbsp toasted pine nuts
- 2 tbsp raisins
- ⅓ cup feta, crumbled
- ½ cup pomegranate seeds
- 2 lemons (juiced, zest grated)
- 8 oz tofu
- 2 tsp oregano
- 2 garlic cloves, minced
- ½ tsp red chili flakes
- 3 tbsp olive oil
- Salt and pepper to taste

Directions:

1. Season the processed cauliflower with salt and transfer to a strainer to drain.
2. Prepare the marinade for tofu by combining 2 tbsp lemon juice, 1.5 tbsp olive oil, minced garlic, chili flakes, oregano, salt and pepper. Coat tofu in the marinade and set aside.
3. Preheat the oven to 450°F.
4. Bake tofu on a baking sheet for 12 minutes.
5. In a salad bowl mix the remaining marinade with onions, cucumber, cauliflower, olives and raisins. Add in the remaining olive oil and grated lemon zest.
6. Top with tofu, pine nuts, feta and pomegranate seeds.

Nutrition: Carbohydrates: 34.1 g Protein: 11.1 g Total sugars: 11.5 g Calories: 328

107. Scallop Caesar Salad

Preparation Time: 5 minutes
Cooking Time: 2 minutes
Servings: 2
Ingredients:

- 8 sea scallops

- 4 cups romaine lettuce
- 2 tsp olive oil
- 3 tbsp Caesar Salad Dressing
- 1 tsp lemon juice
- Salt and pepper to taste

Directions:

1. In a frying pan heat olive oil and cook the scallops in one layer no longer than 2 minutes per both sides. Season with salt and pepper to taste.
2. Arrange lettuce on plates and place scallops on top.
3. Pour over the Caesar dressing and lemon juice.

Nutrition: Carbohydrates: 14 g Protein: 30.7 g Total sugars: 2.2 g Calories: 340 g

108. **Chicken Avocado Salad**

Preparation Time: 30 minutes
Cooking time: 15 minutes
Servings: 4
Ingredients:

- 1 lb chicken breast, cooked, shredded
- 1 avocado, pitted, peeled, sliced
- 2 tomatoes, diced
- 1 cucumber, peeled, sliced
- 1 head lettuce, chopped
- 3 tbsp olive oil
- 2 tbsp lime juice
- 1 tbsp cilantro, chopped
- Salt and pepper to taste

Directions:

1. In a bowl whisk together oil, lime juice, cilantro, salt, and a pinch of pepper.
2. Combine lettuce, tomatoes, cucumber in a salad bowl and toss with half of the dressing.
3. Toss chicken with the remaining dressing and combine with vegetable mixture.
4. Top with avocado.

Nutrition: Carbohydrates: 10 g Protein: 38 g Total sugars: 11.5 g Calories: 380

109. **California Wraps**

Preparation Time: 5 minutes
Cooking Time: 15 minutes
Servings: 4
Ingredients:

- 4 slices turkey breast, cooked
- 4 slices ham, cooked
- 4 lettuce leaves
- 4 slices tomato
- 4 slices avocado
- 1 tsp lime juice
- A handful watercress leaves
- 4 tbsp Ranch dressing, sugar free

Directions:

1. Top a lettuce leaf with turkey slice, ham slice and tomato.
2. In a bowl combine avocado and lime juice and place on top of tomatoes. Top with water cress and dressing.

3. Repeat with the remaining ingredients for 4. Topping each lettuce leaf with a turkey slice, ham slice, tomato and dressing.

Nutrition: Carbohydrates: 4 g Protein: 9 g Total sugars: 0.5 g Calories: 140

110. **Chicken Salad in Cucumber Cups**

Preparation Time: 5 minutes
Cooking Time: 15 minutes
Servings: 4
Ingredients:

- ½ chicken breast, skinless, boiled and shredded
- 2 long cucumbers, cut into 8 thick rounds each, scooped out (won't use in a).
- 1 tsp ginger, minced
- 1 tsp lime zest, grated
- 4 tsp olive oil
- 1 tsp sesame oil
- 1 tsp lime juice
- Salt and pepper to taste

Directions:

1. In a bowl combine lime zest, juice, olive and sesame oils, ginger, season with salt.
2. Toss the chicken with the dressing and fill the cucumber cups with the salad.

Nutrition: Carbohydrates: 4 g Protein: 12 g Total sugars: 0.5 g Calories: 116 g

111. **Sunflower Seeds and Arugula Garden Salad**

Preparation time: 5 minutes
Cooking time: 10 minutes
Servings: 6
Ingredients:

- ¼ tsp black pepper
- ¼ tsp salt
- 1 tsp fresh thyme, chopped
- 2 tbsp. sunflower seeds, toasted
- 2 cups red grapes, halved
- 7 cups baby arugula, loosely packed
- 1 tbsp. coconut oil
- 2 tsp honey
- 3 tbsp. red wine vinegar
- ½ tsp stone-ground mustard

Directions:

1. In a small bowl, whisk together mustard, honey and vinegar. Slowly pour oil as you whisk.
2. In a large salad bowl, mix thyme, seeds, grapes and arugula.
3. Drizzle with dressing and serve.

Nutrition: Calories: 86.7g Protein: 1.6g Carbs: 13.1g Fat: 3.1g.

112. **Supreme Caesar Salad**

Preparation time: 5 minutes
Cooking time: 10 minutes
Servings: 4
Ingredients:

- ¼ cup olive oil
- ¾ cup mayonnaise
- 1 head romaine lettuce, torn into bite sized pieces
- 1 tbsp. lemon juice
- 1 tsp Dijon mustard
- 1 tsp Worcestershire sauce
- 3 cloves garlic, peeled and minced
- 3 cloves garlic, peeled and quartered
- 4 cups day old bread, cubed
- 5 anchovy filets, minced
- 6 tbsp. grated parmesan cheese, divided
- Ground black pepper to taste
- Salt to taste

Directions:

1. In a small bowl, whisk well lemon juice, mustard, Worcestershire sauce, 2 tbsp. parmesan cheese, anchovies, mayonnaise, and minced garlic. Season with pepper and salt to taste. Set aside in the ref.
2. On medium fire, place a large nonstick saucepan and heat oil.
3. Sauté quartered garlic until browned around a minute or two. Remove and discard.
4. Add bread cubes in same pan, sauté until lightly browned. Season with pepper and salt. Transfer to a plate.
5. In large bowl, place lettuce and pour in dressing. Toss well to coat. Top with remaining parmesan cheese.
6. Garnish with bread cubes, serve, and enjoy.

Nutrition: Calories: 443.3g Fat: 32.1g Protein: 11.6g Carbs: 27g

113. **Tabbouleh- Arabian Salad**

Preparation time: 5 minutes
Cooking time: 10 minutes
Servings: 6
Ingredients:

- ¼ cup chopped fresh mint
- 1 2/3 cups boiling water
- 1 cucumber, peeled, seeded and chopped
- 1 cup bulgur
- 1 cup chopped fresh parsley
- 1 cup chopped green onions
- 1 tsp salt
- 1/3 cup lemon juice
- 1/3 cup olive oil
- 3 tomatoes, chopped
- Ground black pepper to taste

Directions:

1. In a large bowl, mix together boiling water and bulgur. Let soak and set aside for an hour while covered.
2. After one hour, toss in cucumber, tomatoes, mint, parsley, onions, lemon juice and oil. Then season with black pepper and salt to taste. Toss well and refrigerate for another hour while covered before serving.

Nutrition: Calories: 185.5g fat: 13.1g Protein: 4.1g Carbs: 12.8g

114. **Tangy Citrus Salad with Grilled Cod**

Preparation time: 5 minutes
Cooking time: 10 minutes
Servings: 2
Ingredients:

- ½ cup orange segments
- ¾ cup chopped red bell pepper
- 1 ½ cups shredded carrot
- 1 ½ cups shredded kohlrabi
- 1 ½ cups shredded spinach
- 1 ½ tbsp. olive oil
- 1 cup grapefruit segments
- 1 cup shredded celery
- 1 tbsp. minced garlic
- 1 tbsp. shredded fresh basil
- 1 tsp black pepper
- 6-oz baked or broiled cod
- Zest and juice of 1 lemon
- Zest and juice of 1 lime
- Zest and juice of 1 orange

Directions:

1. Grease grill grate with cooking spray and preheat to medium high fire. Once grate is hot, grill cod until flaky, around 5 minutes per side.
2. Meanwhile, mix remaining ingredients except for citrus pieces, in a large salad bowl and toss well to combine.
3. To serve, evenly divide salad into two plates, top with ½ of grilled cod and garnish with citrus pieces.

Nutrition: Calories: 381.9g Protein: 22g Carbs: 47.6g Fat: 11.5g.

115. **Thai Salad with Cilantro Lime Dressing**

Preparation time: 10 minutes
Cooking time: 20 minutes
Servings: 2
Ingredients:

- ¼ cup cashews
- ¼ cup fresh mint leaves
- ¼ cup fresh thai basil leaves
- ¼ teaspoon fish sauce
- ½ cup green papaya, julienned
- ½ teaspoon honey
- 1 head green leaf lettuce, chopped
- 1 loose handful fresh cilantro
- 1 tablespoon lime juice
- 1 teaspoon coconut amines
- 3 tablespoons olive oil
- 3 tangerines, peeled and segmented

Directions:

1. Prepare the lime cilantro dressing by mixing honey, fresh cilantro, fish sauce, coconut amines, lime juice and oil in a mixing bowl. Mix then set aside.
2. Prepare the salad by mixing the remaining six ingredients. Toss everything to distribute the ingredients.
3. Toss the salad dressing into the vegetables.
4. Serve chilled.

Nutrition: Calories: 649.8g fat: 57.4 g Protein: 7.5 g Carbs: 25.8 g.

116. Truffle Oil, Mushrooms and Cauliflower Salad

Preparation time: 10 minutes
Cooking time: 25 minutes
Servings: 4
Ingredients:

- ¼ tsp fresh ground black pepper
- ¼ tsp Salt
- 1 ½ oz grate pecorino-romano cheese, divide
- 1 15-oz bpa free can unsalted cannellini beans, drained and rinsed (try Eden organic cannellini beans)
- 1 cup low-sodium chicken broth
- 1 large head cauliflower, chopped into florets
- 1 yellow onion, chopped
- 1/3 cup chopped fresh flat leaf parsley leaves
- 2 tbsp. fresh lemon juice
- 3 cloves garlic, minced
- 4 tsp truffle oil
- 8 oz. cremini mushrooms, sliced
- Olive oil cooking spray

Directions:

1. Divide cauliflower in 3 batches and process in a food processor until the size of a rice grain. Repeat until all batches are done.
2. Next blend together broth and beans for a minute or until smooth.
3. On medium low fire, place a large pan and grease with cooking spray.
4. Add onions and mushrooms; stir-fry until liquid is almost gone around 5-7 minutes.
5. Add pepper, salt and garlic. Cook for a minute more.
6. Increase fire to medium high and add lemon juice. Cook and stir for a minute or until liquid has evaporated.
7. Add pureed beans and bring to a simmer. Once simmering, add cauliflower and mix well. Cover, reduce fire to medium, and stir occasionally as you cook cauliflower until tender, around 8-10 minutes.
8. Once cauliflower is tender, turn off heat.
9. Add truffle oil, parsley and ¾ oz cheese. Mix well.
10. 1 evenly divide on to bowls, top with remaining cheese and serve.

Nutrition: Calories: 506.1g Protein: 19.3g Carbs: 76.4g Fat: 13.7g

117. Tuna Avocado Salad

Preparation time: 5 minutes

Cooking time: 0 minutes
Servings: 4
Ingredients:

- 1 avocado, pit removed and sliced
- 1 lemon, juiced
- 1 tablespoon chopped onion
- 5 ounces cooked or canned tuna
- Salt and pepper to taste

Directions:

1. In a mixing bowl, combine the avocado and lime juice. Mash the avocado and add the tuna.
2. Season with salt and pepper to taste.
3. Serve chilled.

Nutrition: Calories: 695.5g Fat: 50.7 g Protein: 41.5 g Carbs: 18.3 g

118. Tuna-Mediterranean Salad

Preparation time: 15 minutes
Cooking time: 0 minutes
Servings: 6
Ingredients:

- ¼ cup chopped pitted ripe olives
- ¼ cup drained and chopped roasted red peppers
- ¼ cup mayonnaise dressing with olive oil
- 1 tbsp. small capers, rinsed and drained
- 2 green onions, sliced
- 2 pcs of 6 oz. cans of tuna, drained and flaked
- 6 slices whole wheat bread optional
- Salad greens like lettuce optional

Directions:

1. With the exception of salad greens or bread, mix together all of the ingredients: in a bowl. If desired, you can arrange it on top of salad greens or serve with bread

Nutrition: Calories: 197.1g Protein: 6.9g Fat: 5.7g Carbs: 16.3g

119. Southwestern Bean-And-Pepper Salad

Preparation Time: 6 minutes
Cooking Time: 0 minutes
Servings: 4
Ingredients:

- 1 (15-ounce) can pinto beans, drained and rinsed
- 2 bell peppers, cored and chopped
- 1 cup corn kernels (cut from 1 to 2 ears or frozen and thawed)
- Salt
- Freshly ground black pepper
- Juice of 2 limes
- 1 tablespoon olive oil
- 1 avocado, chopped

Directions:

1. In a large bowl, combine beans, peppers, corn, salt, and pepper. Squeeze fresh lime juice to taste and stir in olive oil. Let the mixture stand in the refrigerator for 30 minutes.
2. Add avocado just before serving.

3. Budget-saver tip avocado prices can vary dramatically depending on their availability. In addition, while avocado in your salad can really add flavor and satiety, for an equally delicious salad you could add a cup of cooked and chopped sweet potatoes with 1 to 2 tablespoons of sunflower seeds.

Nutrition: Total calories: 245 Total fat: 11g Saturated fat: 2g Cholesterol: 0mg Sodium: 97mg Potassium: 380mg Total carbohydrate: 32g Fiber: 10g Sugars: 4g Protein: 8g.

120. Cauliflower Mashed "Potatoes"

Preparation Time: 10 minutes
Cooking Time: 10 minutes
Servings: 4
Ingredients:

- 16 cups water (enough to cover cauliflower)
- 1 head cauliflower (about 3 pounds), trimmed and cut into florets
- 4 garlic cloves
- 1 tablespoon olive oil
- ¼ teaspoon salt
- ⅛ teaspoon freshly ground black pepper
- 2 teaspoons dried parsley

Directions:

1. Bring a large pot of water to a boil. Add the cauliflower and garlic. Cook for about 10 minutes or until the cauliflower is fork tender. Drain, return it back to the hot pan, and let it stand for 2 to 3 minutes with the lid on.
2. Transfer the cauliflower and garlic to a food processor or blender. Add the olive oil, salt, pepper, and purée until smooth.
3. Taste and adjust the salt and pepper. Remove to a serving bowl, add the parsley, and mix until combined.
4. Garnish with additional olive oil, if desired. Serve immediately.
5. Ingredient tip if you don't have a food processor or blender, you can make this dish just as you would traditional mashed potatoes by using a potato masher or hand blender.

Nutrition: Total calories: 87g Total fat: 4g Saturated fat: 1g Cholesterol: 0mg Sodium: 210mg Potassium: 654mg Total carbohydrate: 12g Fiber: 5g Sugars: 0g Protein: 4g

121. Roasted Brussels sprouts

Preparation time: 5 minutes
Cooking time: 20 minutes
Servings: 4
Ingredients:

- 1½ pounds Brussels sprouts, trimmed and halved
- 2 tablespoons olive oil
- ¼ teaspoon salt
- ½ teaspoon freshly ground black pepper

Directions:

1. Preheat the oven to 400°f.
2. Combine the Brussels sprouts and olive oil in a large mixing bowl and toss until they are evenly coated.
3. Turn the Brussels sprouts out onto a large baking sheet and flip them over so they are cut-side down with the flat part touching the baking sheet. Sprinkle with salt and pepper.
4. Bake for 20 to 30 minutes or until the Brussels sprouts are lightly charred and crisp on the outside and toasted on the bottom. The outer leaves will be extra dark, too.
5. Serve immediately.
6. Ingredient tip when choosing Brussels sprouts, look for bright-green heads that are firm and heavy for their size. The leaves should be tightly packed. Avoid sprouts with yellowing leaves—a sign of age—or black spots—which means they could have fungus.

Nutrition: Total calories: 134 Total fat: 8g Saturated fat: 1g Cholesterol: 0mg Sodium: 189mg Potassium: 665mg Total carbohydrate: 15g Fiber: 7g; Sugars: 4g Protein: 6g

122. Green Salad with Blackberries, Goat Cheese, and Sweet Potatoes

Preparation Time: 15 minutes
Cooking Time: 20 minutes
Servings: 4
Ingredients:
FOR THE VINAIGRETTE

- 1 pint blackberries
- 2 tablespoons red wine vinegar
- 1 tablespoon honey
- 3 tablespoons extra-virgin olive oil
- ¼ teaspoon salt
- Freshly ground black pepper

FOR THE SALAD

- 1 sweet potato, cubed
- 1 teaspoon extra-virgin olive oil
- 8 cups salad greens (baby spinach, spicy greens, romaine)
- ½ red onion, sliced
- ¼ cup crumbled goat cheese

Directions:

1. TO MAKE THE VINAIGRETTE
2. In a blender jar, combine the blackberries, vinegar, honey, oil, salt, and pepper, and process until smooth. Set aside.
3. TO MAKE THE SALAD
4. Preheat the oven to 425°F. Line a baking sheet with parchment paper.
5. In a medium mixing bowl, toss the sweet potato with the olive oil. Transfer to the Preparebaking sheet and roast for 20 minutes, stirring once halfway through, until tender. Remove and cool for a few minutes.
6. 3.In a large bowl, toss the greens with the red onion and cooled sweet potato, and drizzle with the

vinaigrette. Serve topped with 1 tablespoon of goat cheese per serving.

Nutrition: Calories: 196 Total Fat: 12g Protein: 3g Carbohydrates: 21g Sugars: 10g Fiber: 6g Sodium: 184mg

123. Warm Barley and Squash Salad with Balsamic Vinaigrette

Preparation Time: 20 minutes
Cooking Time: 40 minutes
Servings: 8
Ingredients:

- 1 small butternut squash
- 3 teaspoons plus 2 tablespoons extra-virgin olive oil, divided
- 2 cups broccoli florets
- 1 cup pearl barley
- 1 cup toasted chopped walnuts
- 2 cups baby kale
- ½ red onion, sliced
- 2 tablespoons balsamic vinegar
- 2 garlic cloves, minced
- ½ teaspoon salt
- ¼ teaspoon freshly ground black pepper

Directions:

1. Preheat the oven to 400°F. Line a baking sheet with parchment paper.
2. Peel and seed the squash, and cut it into dice. In a large bowl, toss the squash with 2 teaspoons of olive oil. Transfer to the prepare baking sheet and roast for 20 minutes.
3. While the squash is roasting, toss the broccoli in the same bowl with 1 teaspoon of olive oil. After 20 minutes, flip the squash and push it to one side of the baking sheet. Add the broccoli to the other side and continue to roast for 20 more minutes until tender.
4. While the veggies are roasting, in a medium pot, cover the barley with several inches of water. Bring to a boil, then reduce the heat, cover, and simmer for 30 minutes until tender. Drain and rinse.
5. Transfer the barley to a large bowl, and toss with the cooked squash and broccoli, walnuts, kale, and onion.
6. In a small bowl, mix the remaining 2 tablespoons of olive oil, balsamic vinegar, garlic, salt, and pepper. Toss the salad with the dressing and serve.

Nutrition: Calories: 274 Total Fat: 15g Protein: 6g Carbohydrates: 32g Sugars: 3g Fiber: 7g Sodium: 144mg

124. Salmon, Quinoa, and Avocado Salad

Preparation Time: 15 minutes
Cooking Time: 20 minutes
Servings: 4
Ingredients:

- ½ cup quinoa
- 1 cup water
- 4 (4-ounce) salmon fillets
- 1-pound asparagus, trimmed
- 1 teaspoon extra-virgin olive oil, plus 2 tablespoons
- ½ teaspoon salt, divided
- ½ teaspoon freshly ground black pepper, divided
- ¼ teaspoon red pepper flakes
- 1 avocado, chopped
- ¼ cup chopped scallions, both white and green parts
- ¼ cup chopped fresh cilantro
- 1 tablespoon minced fresh oregano
- Juice of 1 lime

Directions:

1. In a small pot, combine the quinoa and water, and bring to a boil over medium-high heat. Cover, reduce the heat, and simmer for 15 minutes.
2. Preheat the oven to 425°F. Line a large baking sheet with parchment paper.
3. Arrange the salmon on one side of the prepared baking sheet. Toss the asparagus with 1 teaspoon of olive oil, and arrange on the other side of the baking sheet. Season the salmon and asparagus with ¼ teaspoon of salt, ¼ teaspoon of pepper, and the red pepper flakes. Roast for 12 minutes until browned and cooked through.
4. While the fish and asparagus are cooking, in a large mixing bowl, gently toss the cooked quinoa, avocado, scallions, cilantro, and oregano. Add the remaining 2 tablespoons of olive oil and the lime juice, and season with the remaining ¼ teaspoon of salt and ¼ teaspoon of pepper.
5. Break the salmon into pieces, removing the skin and any bones, and chop the asparagus into bite-sized pieces. Fold into the quinoa and serve warm or at room temperature.

Nutrition: Calories: 397 Total Fat: 22g Protein: 29g Carbohydrates: 23g Sugars: 3g Fiber: 8g Sodium: 292mg

125. Cucumber, Tomato, and Avocado Salad

Preparation Time: 10 minutes
Cooking Time: 0 min
Servings: 4
Ingredients:

- 1 cup cherry tomatoes, halved
- 1 large cucumber, chopped
- 1 small red onion, thinly sliced
- 1 avocado, diced
- 2 tablespoons chopped fresh dill
- 2 tablespoons extra-virgin olive oil
- Juice of 1 lemon
- ¼ teaspoon salt
- ¼ teaspoon freshly ground black pepper

Directions

1. In a large mixing bowl, combine the tomatoes, cucumber, onion, avocado, and dill.
2. In a small bowl, combine the oil, lemon juice, salt, and pepper, and mix well.
3. Drizzle the dressing over the vegetables and toss to combine. Serve.

Nutrition: Calories: 151 Total Fat: 12g Protein: 2g Carbohydrates: 11g Sugars: 4g Fiber: 4g Sodium: 128mg

126. Cabbage Slaw Salad

Preparation Time: 15 minutes
Cooking Time: 0 min
Servings: 6
Ingredients:

- 2 cups finely chopped green cabbage
- 2 cups finely chopped red cabbage
- 2 cups grated carrots
- 3 scallions, both white and green parts, sliced
- 2 tablespoons extra-virgin olive oil
- 2 tablespoons rice vinegar
- 1 teaspoon honey
- 1 garlic clove, minced
- ¼ teaspoon salt

Directions:

1. In a large bowl, toss together the green and red cabbage, carrots, and scallions.
2. In a small bowl, whisk together the oil, vinegar, honey, garlic, and salt.
3. Pour the dressing over the veggies and mix to thoroughly combine.
4. Serve immediately, or cover and chill for several hours before serving.

Nutrition: Calories: 80 Total Fat: 5g Protein: 1g Carbohydrates: 10g Sugars: 6g Fiber: 3g Sodium: 126mg

127. Winter Chicken and Citrus Salad

Preparation Time: 10 minutes
Cooking Time: 0 min
Servings: 4
Ingredients:

- 4 cups baby spinach
- 2 tablespoons extra-virgin olive oil
- 1 tablespoon freshly squeezed lemon juice
- ⅛ teaspoon salt
- Freshly ground black pepper
- 2 cups chopped cooked chicken
- 2 mandarin oranges, peeled and sectioned
- ½ peeled grapefruit, sectioned
- ¼ cup sliced almonds

Directions:

1. In a large mixing bowl, toss the spinach with the olive oil, lemon juice, salt, and pepper.
2. Add the chicken, oranges, grapefruit, and almonds to the bowl. Toss gently.
3. Arrange on 4 plates and serve.

Nutrition: Calories: 249 Total Fat: 12g Protein: 24g Carbohydrates: 11g Sugars: 7g Fiber: 3g Sodium: 135mg

128. Blueberry and Chicken Salad on a Bed of Greens

Preparation Time: 10 minutes
Cooking Time: 0 min
Servings: 4
Ingredients:

- 2 cups chopped cooked chicken
- 1 cup fresh blueberries
- ¼ cup finely chopped almonds
- 1 celery stalk, finely chopped
- ¼ cup finely chopped red onion
- 1 tablespoon chopped fresh basil
- 1 tablespoon chopped fresh cilantro
- ½ cup plain, nonfat Greek yogurt or vegan mayonnaise
- ¼ teaspoon salt
- ¼ teaspoon freshly ground black pepper
- 8 cups salad greens (baby spinach, spicy greens, romaine)

Directions:

1. In a large mixing bowl, combine the chicken, blueberries, almonds, celery, onion, basil, and cilantro. Toss gently to mix.
2. In a small bowl, combine the yogurt, salt, and pepper. Add to the chicken salad and stir to combine.
3. Arrange 2 cups of salad greens on each of 4 plates and divide the chicken salad among the plates to serve.

Nutrition: Calories: 207 Total Fat: 6g Protein: 28g Carbohydrates: 11g Sugars: 6g Fiber: 3g Sodium: 235mg

129. Cauliflower & Apple Salad

Preparation Time: 25 minutes
Cooking Time: 0 minutes
Servings: 4
Ingredients:

- 3 Cups Cauliflower, Chopped into Florets
- 2 Cups Baby Kale
- 1 Sweet Apple, Cored & Chopped
- ¼ Cup Basil, Fresh & Chopped
- ¼ Cup Mint, Fresh & Chopped
- ¼ Cup Parsley, Fresh & Chopped
- 1/3 Cup Scallions, Sliced Thin
- 2 Tablespoons Yellow Raisins
- 1 Tablespoon Sun Dried Tomatoes, Chopped
- ½ Cup Miso Dressing, Optional
- ¼ Cup Roasted Pumpkin Seeds, Optional

Directions:

1. Combine everything together, tossing before serving.
2. Interesting Facts: This vegetable is an extremely high source of vitamin A, vitamin B1, B2 and B3.

Nutrition: Calories: 198 Protein: 7 Grams Fat: 8 Grams Carbs: 32 Grams

130. Corn & Black Bean Salad

Preparation Time: 10 minutes
Cooking Time: 0 minutes
Servings: 6
Ingredients:

- ¼ Cup Cilantro, Fresh & Chopped
- 1 Can Corn, Drained (10 Ounces)
- 1/8 Cup Red Onion, Chopped

- 1 Can Black Beans, Drained (15 Ounces)
- 1 Tomato, Chopped
- 3 Tablespoons Lemon Juice, Fresh
- 2 Tablespoons Olive Oil
- Sea Salt & Black Pepper to Taste

Directions:
1. Mix everything together, and then refrigerates until cool. Serve cold.
2. Interesting Facts: Whole corn is a fantastic source of phosphorus, magnesium, and B vitamins. It also promotes healthy digestion and contains heart-healthy antioxidants. It is important to seek out organic corn in order to bypass all of the genetically modified product that is out on the market.

Nutrition: Calories: 159 Protein: 6.4 Grams Fat: 5.6 Grams Carbs: 23.7 Grams

131. <u>Spinach & Orange Salad</u>

Preparation Time: 15 minutes
Cooking Time: 0 minutes
Servings: 6
Ingredients:
- ¼ -1/3 Cup Vegan Dressing
- 3 Oranges, Medium, Peeled, Seeded & Sectioned
- ¾ lb. Spinach, Fresh & Torn
- 1 Red Onion, Medium, Sliced & Separated into Rings

Directions:
1. Toss everything together, and serve with dressing.
2. Interesting Facts: Spinach is one of the most superb green veggies out there. Each serving is packed with 3 grams of protein and is a highly encouraged component of the plant-based diet.

Nutrition: Calories: 99 Protein: 2.5 Grams Fat: 5 Grams Carbs: 13.1 Grams

132. <u>Red Pepper & Broccoli Salad</u>

Preparation Time: 15 minutes
Cooking Time: 0 minutes
Servings: 2
Ingredients:
- Ounces Lettuce Salad Mix
- 1 Head Broccoli, Chopped into Florets
- 1 Red Pepper, Seeded & Chopped
- Dressing:
- 3 Tablespoons White Wine Vinegar
- 1 Teaspoon Dijon Mustard
- 1 Clove Garlic, Peeled & Chopped Fine
- ½ Teaspoon Black Pepper
- ½ Teaspoon Sea Salt, Fine
- 2 Tablespoons Olive Oil
- 1 Tablespoon Parsley, Chopped

Directions:
1. In boiling water, drain the broccoli it on a paper towel.
2. Whisk together all dressing ingredients.
3. Toss ingredients together before serving.
4. Interesting Facts: This oil is the main source of dietary fat in a variety of diets. It contains many

vitamins and minerals that play a part in reducing the risk of stroke and lowers cholesterol and high blood pressure and can also aid in weight loss. It is best consumed cold, as when it is heated it can lose some of its nutritive properties (although it is still great to cook with: extra virgin is best), many recommend taking a shot of cold oil olive daily! Bonus: if you don't like the taste or texture add a shot to your smoothie.

Nutrition: Calories: 185 Protein: 4 Grams Fat: 14 Grams Carbs: 8 Grams

133. <u>Lentil Potato Salad</u>

Preparation Time: 35 minutes
Cooking Time: 25 minutes
Servings: 2
Ingredients:
- ½ Cup Beluga Lentils
- 8 Fingerling Potatoes
- 1 Cup Scallions, Sliced Thin
- ¼ Cup Cherry Tomatoes, Halved
- ¼ Cup Lemon Vinaigrette
- Sea Salt & Black Pepper to Taste

Directions:
1. Bring two cups of water to simmer in a pot, adding your lentils. Cook for twenty to twenty-five minutes, and then drain. Your lentils should be tender.
2. Reduce to a simmer, cooking for fifteen minutes, and then drain. Halve your potatoes once they're cool enough to touch.
3. Put your lentils on a serving plate, and then top with scallions, potatoes and tomatoes. Drizzle with your vinaigrette, and season with salt and pepper.
4. Interesting Facts: Lemons are popularly known as harboring loads of Vitamin C, but are also excellent sources of folate, fiber, and antioxidants. Bonus: Helps lower cholesterol. Double Bonus: Reduces risk of cancer and high blood pressure.

Nutrition: Calories: 400 Protein: 7 Grams Fat: 26 Grams Carbs: 39 Grams

134. <u>Black Bean & Corn Salad with Avocado</u>

Preparation Time: 20 minutes
Cooking Time: 15 minutes
Servings: 6
Ingredients:
- 1 and 1/2 cups corn kernels, cooked & frozen or canned
- 1/2 cup olive oil
- 1 minced clove garlic
- 1/3 cup lime juice, fresh
- 1 avocado (peeled, pitted & diced)
- 1/8 tsp. cayenne pepper
- 2 cans black beans, (approximately 15 oz.)
- 6 thinly sliced green onions
- 1/2 cup chopped cilantro, fresh
- 2 chopped tomatoes

- 1 chopped red bell pepper
- Chili powder
- 1/2 tsp. salt

Directions:
1. In a small jar, place the olive oil, lime juice, garlic, cayenne, and salt.
2. Cover with lid; shake until all the ingredients under the jar are mixed well.
3. Toss the green onions, corn, beans, bell pepper, avocado, tomatoes, and cilantro together in a large bowl or plastic container with a cover.
4. Shake the lime dressing for a second time and transfer it over the salad ingredients.
5. Stir salad to coat the beans and vegetables with the dressing; cover & refrigerate.
6. To blend the flavors completely, let this sit a moment or two.
7. Remove the container from the refrigerator from time to time; turn upside down & back gently a couple of times to reorganize the dressing.

Nutrition: 448 Calories 24.3 g Total Fat 0 mg Cholesterol 50.8 g Total Carbohydrate 14.3 g Dietary Fiber 13.2 g Protein

135. Summer Chickpea Salad
Preparation Time: 15 minutes
Cooking Time: 15 minutes
Servings: 4
Ingredients:
- 1 ½ Cups Cherry Tomatoes, Halved
- 1 Cup English Cucumber, Slices
- 1 Cup Chickpeas, Canned, Unsalted, Drained & Rinsed
- ¼ Cup Red Onion, Slivered
- 2 Tablespoon Olive Oil
- 1 ½ Tablespoons Lemon Juice, Fresh
- 1 ½ Tablespoons Lemon Juice, Fresh
- Sea Salt & Black Pepper to Taste

Directions:
1. Mix everything together, and toss to combine before serving.

Nutrition: Calories: 145 Protein: 4 Grams Fat: 7.5 Grams Carbs: 16 Grams

136. Edamame Salad
Preparation Time: 15 minutes
Cooking Time: 0 minutes
Servings: 1
Ingredients:
- ¼ Cup Red Onion, Chopped
- 1 Cup Corn Kernels, Fresh
- 1 Cup Edamame Beans, Shelled & Thawed
- 1 Red Bell Pepper, Chopped
- 2-3 Tablespoons Lime Juice, Fresh
- 5-6 Basil Leaves, Fresh & Sliced
- 5-6 Mint Leaves, Fresh & Sliced
- Sea Salt & Black Pepper to Taste

Directions:

1. Place everything into a Mason jar, and then seal the jar tightly. Shake well before serving.
2. Interesting Facts: Whole corn is a fantastic source of phosphorus, magnesium, and B vitamins. It also promotes healthy digestion and contains heart-healthy antioxidants. It is important to seek out organic corn in order to bypass all of the genetically modified product that is out on the market.

Nutrition: Calories: 299 Protein: 20 Grams Fat: 9 Grams Carbs: 38 Grams

137. Fruity Kale Salad
Preparation Time: 30 minutes
Cooking Time: 0 minutes
Servings: 4
Ingredients:
- Salad:
- 10 Ounces Baby Kale
- ½ Cup Pomegranate Arils
- 1 Tablespoon Olive Oil
- 1 Apple, Sliced
- Dressing:
- 3 Tablespoons Apple Cider Vinegar
- 3 Tablespoons Olive Oil
- 1 Tablespoon Tahini Sauce (Optional)
- Sea Salt & Black Pepper to Taste

Directions:
1. Wash and dry the kale. If kale is too expensive, you can also use lettuce, arugula or spinach. Take the stems out, and chop it.
2. Combine all of your salad ingredients together.
3. Combine all of your dressing ingredients together before drizzling it over the salad to serve.

Nutrition: Calories: 220 Protein: 4 Grams Fat: 17 Grams Carbs: 16 Grams

138. Olive & Fennel Salad
Preparation Time: 5 minutes
Cooking Time: 0 minutes
Servings: 3
Ingredients:
- 6 Tablespoons Olive Oil
- 3 Fennel Bulbs, Trimmed, Cored & Quartered
- 2 Tablespoons Parsley, Fresh & Chopped
- 1 Lemon, Juiced & Zested
- 12 Black Olives
- Sea Salt & Black Pepper to Taste

Directions:
1. Grease your baking dish, and then place your fennel in it. Make sure the cut side is up.
2. Mix your lemon zest, lemon juice, salt, pepper and oil, pouring it over your fennel.
3. Sprinkle your olives over it, and bake at 400.
4. Serve with parsley.
5. Interesting Facts: This oil is the main source of dietary fat in a variety of diets. It contains many vitamins and minerals that play a part in reducing the risk of stroke and lowers cholesterol and high blood pressure and can also aid in weight loss. It is best consumed cold, as when it is heated it can lose

some of its nutritive properties (although it is still great to cook with: extra virgin is best), many recommend taking a shot of cold oil olive daily! Bonus: if you don't like the taste or texture add a shot to your smoothie

Nutrition: Calories: 331 Protein: 3 Grams Fat: 29 Grams Carbs: 15 Grams

139. **Tomato Gazpacho**

Preparation Time: 2 hours and 25 minutes
Cooking Time: 0 minutes
Servings: 6
Ingredients:

- 2 Tablespoons + 1 Teaspoon Red Wine Vinegar, Divided
- ½ Teaspoon Pepper
- 1 Teaspoon Sea Salt
- 1 Avocado,
- ¼ Cup Basil, Fresh & Chopped
- 3 Tablespoons + 2 Teaspoons Olive Oil, Divided
- 1 Clove Garlic, crushed
- 1 Red Bell Pepper, Sliced & Seeded
- 1 Cucumber, Chunked
- 2 ½ lbs. Large Tomatoes, Cored & Chopped

Directions:

1. Place half of your cucumber, bell pepper, and ¼ cup of each tomato in a bowl, covering. Set it in the fried.
2. Puree your remaining tomatoes, cucumber and bell pepper with garlic, three tablespoons oil, two tablespoons of vinegar, sea salt and black pepper into a blender, blending until smooth. Transfer it to a bowl, and chill for two hours.
3. Chop the avocado, adding it to your chopped vegetables, adding your remaining oil, vinegar, salt, pepper and basil.
4. Ladle your tomato puree mixture into bowls, and serve with chopped vegetables as a salad.

Nutrition: Calories: 181 Protein: 3 Grams Fat: 14 Grams Carbs: 14 Grams

140. **Snow White Salad**

Preparation Time: 10 minutes
Cooking Time: 5 minutes
Servings: 4
Ingredients:

- 1 large or two small cucumbers -fresh or pickled
- 4 cups of plain yogurt
- ½ cup of crushed walnuts
- 2-3 cloves garlic, crushed
- ½ bunch of dill
- 3 tbsp sunflower oil
- salt, to taste

Directions:

1. Strain the yogurt in a piece of cheesecloth or a clean white dishtowel. You can suspend it over a bowl or the sink.
2. Peel and dice the cucumbers, place in a large bowl. Add the crushed walnuts and the crushed garlic, the

oil and the finely chopped dill. Scoop the drained yogurt into the bowl and stir well.

3. Add salt to the taste, cover with cling film, and put in the fridge for at least an hour so the flavors can mix well.

Nutrition: Calories: 523; Total fat: 50g; Total carbs: 9g; Fiber: 4g; Sugar: 2g; Protein: 13g; Sodium: 366mg

141. **Green Salad**

Preparation Time: 10 minutes
Cooking Time: 5 minutes
Servings: 4
Ingredients:

- one head of green lettuce, washed and drained
- 1 cucumber, sliced
- a bunch of radishes, sliced
- a bunch of spring onions, finely cut
- the juice of half a lemon or 2 tbsp of white wine vinegar
- 3 tbsp sunflower or olive oil
- salt, to taste

Directions:

1. Cut the lettuce into thin strips. Slice the cucumber and the radishes as thinly as possible and chop the spring onions.
2. Mix all the salad ingredients in a large salad bowl; add the lemon juice and oil and season with salt to taste.

Nutrition: Calories: 242; Total fat: 9g; Total carbs: 35g; Fiber: 10g; Sugar: 8g; Protein: 9g; Sodium: 688mg

142. **Roasted Eggplant and Pepper Dip**

Preparation Time: 10 minutes
Cooking Time: 5 minutes
Servings: 4
Ingredients:

- 2 medium eggplants
- 2 red or green bell peppers
- 2 tomatoes
- 3 cloves garlic, crushed
- fresh parsley
- 1-2 tbsp red wine vinegar
- olive oil, as needed
- salt, pepper

Directions:

1. Wash and dry the vegetables. Prick the skin of the eggplants. Bake the eggplants, tomatoes and peppers in a pre-heated oven at 480 F for about 40 minutes, until the skins are pretty burnt. Take out of the oven and leave in a covered container for about 10 minutes.
2. Peel the skins off and drain well the extra juices. De-seed the peppers. Cut all the vegetables into small pieces. Add the garlic and mix well with a fork or in a food processor.
3. Add the olive oil, vinegar and salt to taste. Stir again. Serve cold and sprinkled with parsley.

Nutrition: Calories: 476; Total fat: 40g; Total carbs: 26g; Fiber: 11g; Sugar: 10g; Protein: 9g; Sodium: 655mg

143. Russian Salad

Preparation Time: 15 minutes
Cooking Time: 5 minutes
Servings: 4
Ingredients:
- 3 potatoes
- 2 carrots
- 1 cup green peas, cooked, drained
- 1 cup mayonnaise
- 5-6 pickled gherkins, chopped
- salt, to taste
- 6-7 black olives, to serve

Directions:
1. Boil the potatoes and carrots, then chop into small cubes. Put everything, except for the mayonnaise, in a serving bowl and mix. Add salt to taste, then stir in the mayonnaise.
2. Garnish with parsley and olives. Serve cold.

Nutrition: Calories: 326; Total fat: 24g; Total carbs: 22g; Fiber: 4g; Sugar: 7g; Protein: 8g; Sodium: 573mg

144. Fried Zucchinis with Yogurt Sauce

Preparation Time: 10 minutes
Cooking Time: 5 minutes
Servings: 4
Ingredients:
- 4 zucchinis medium size
- 1 ½ cup yogurt
- 3 cloves garlic, crushed
- a bunch of fresh dill, chopped
- 1 cup all-purpose flour
- salt, to taste

Directions:
1. Start by combining the garlic and chopped dill with the yogurt in a bowl. Add salt to taste and put in the fridge.
2. Wash and peel the zucchinis, and cut them in thin diagonal slices or in rings 0.20 inch thick. Salt and leave them in a suitable bowl placing it inclined to drain away the juices.
3. Coat the zucchinis with flour, then fry turning on both sides until they are golden-brown (about 3 minutes on each side). Transfer to paper towels and pat dry. Serve the zucchinis hot or cold, with garlic yogurt on the side.

Nutrition: Calories: 499; Total fat: 41g; Total carbs: 26g; Fiber: 8g; Sugar: 9g; Protein: 12g; Sodium: 859mg

145. Lyutenitsa-Bulgarian Tomato Dip

Preparation Time: 10 minutes
Cooking Time: 5 minutes
Servings: 4
Ingredients:
- 5 lbs red peppers
- 4 lbs roma tomatoes
- 3 lb eggplant
- 2 lb carrots
- 6-7 garlic cloves, pressed
- 1/3 cup sugar
- 3-4 tsp salt
- 2/3 cup sunflower oil
- Black pepper (optional)

Directions:
1. Wash and roast the eggplants and peppers in a pre-heated oven at 480 F until the skins are pretty burnt. Take out of the oven and leave in a covered container for about 5 minutes. Peel the skins off and drain well the extra juices. Blend in a blender.
2. Wash the tomatoes well, cut and blend on the lower setting of a blender until they are still chunky, but not too much.
3. Boil the carrots.
4. Combine all vegetables in a large pot. Add in garlic, sugar, salt and oil and boil, stirring often, on medium-high heat for about 3-4 hours or until the liquid evaporates and the lyutenitsa thickens. You can also use the oven and bake the lyutenitsa in it.
5. Check whether the lyutenitsa is done by putting a spoonful on a clean, dry plate - if there is a large "watery ring" around the thicker mixture, it's not done yet.
6. When done, ladle into hot jars. Flip upside down or process 10 minutes in boiling water.

Nutrition: Calories: 306; Total fat: 20g; Total carbs: 24g; Fiber: 6g; Sugar: 7g; Protein: 11g; Sodium: 706mg

146. Potato Salad

Preparation Time: 10 minutes
Cooking Time: 5 minutes
Servings: 4
Ingredients:
- 4-5 large potatoes
- 2-3 spring onions, finely chopped
- juice of ½ a lemon
- 5 tbsp sunflower or olive oil
- salt and pepper, to taste
- fresh parsley

Directions:
1. Peel and boil the potatoes for about 20-25 minutes, drain and leave to cool.
2. In a salad bowl add the finely chopped spring onions, the lemon juice, salt, pepper and olive oil, and mix gently. Cut the potatoes into cubes and add to the salad bowl. Gently mix, sprinkle with parsley. Serve cold.

Nutrition: Calories: 238; Total fat: 1g;Total carbs: 46g; Fiber: 7g; Sugar: 29g; Protein: 16g; Sodium: 15mg

147. Garlic Dip

Preparation Time: 15 minutes
Cooking Time: 10 minutes
Servings: 4
Ingredients:
- 2 potatoes
- 6-7 garlic cloves, finely chopped

- 1 cup finely chopped walnuts
- ½ cup extra virgin olive oil
- 1/4 cup red wine vinegar

Directions:

1. Combine boiled and peeled potatoes, chopped garlic, walnuts and salt in a blender. Puree for 30 seconds until everything is well blended. Slowly pour in oil and vinegar, alternating between them.
2. Continue pureeing for about 3 minutes until mixture is a smooth paste a little looser than mashed potatoes in texture.

Nutrition: Calories: 291; Total fat: 21g; Total carbs: 21g; Fiber: 5g; Sugar: 14g; Protein: 10g; Sodium: 242mg

148. White Bean Salad

Preparation Time: 5 minutes
Cooking Time: 10 minutes
Servings: 2
Ingredients:

- 1 cup white beans
- 1 onion
- 3 tbsp white vinegar
- a bunch of fresh parsley
- salt and black pepper

Directions:

1. Wash the beans and soak them in cold water to swell overnight. Cook in the same water with the peeled onion. When tender, drain and put into a deeper bowl. Remove the onion.
2. Mix well oil, vinegar, salt and pepper. Pour over still warm beans, leave to cool about 30-40 minutes.
3. Chop the onion and the parsley, add to the beans, mix and leave to cool for at least 40 minutes. Serve cold.

Nutrition: Calories: 450; Total fat: 13g; Total carbs: 68g;Fiber: 12g; Sugar: 7g; Protein: 17g; Sodium: 791mg

MEAT RECIPE

149. Nut-Stuffed Pork Chops

Preparation time: 20 minutes
Cooking time: 30 minutes
Servings: 4
Ingredients:

- 3 ounces' goat cheese
- ½ cup chopped walnuts
- ¼ cup toasted chopped almonds
- 1 teaspoon chopped fresh thyme
- 4 center-cut pork chops, butterflied
- Sea salt
- Freshly ground black pepper
- 2 tablespoons olive oil

Directions:

1. Preheat the oven to 400°F.
2. In a small bowl, make the filling by stirring together the goat cheese, walnuts, almonds, and thyme until well mixed.
3. Season the pork chops inside and outside with salt and pepper. Stuff each chop, pushing the filling to the bottom of the cut section. Secure the stuffing with toothpicks through the meat.
4. Place a large skillet over medium-high heat and add the olive oil. Pan sear the pork chops until they're browned on each side, about 10 minutes in total.
5. Transfer the pork chops to a baking dish and roast the chops in the oven until cooked through, about 20 minutes.
6. Serve after removing the toothpicks.

Nutrition: Calories: 481 Fat: 38g Protein: 29g Carbs: 5g Fiber: 3g Net Carbs: 2g Fat 70%/Protein 25%/Carbs 5%

150. Roasted Pork Loin with Grainy Mustard Sauce

Preparation time: 10 minutes
Cooking time: 70 minutes
Servings: 8
Ingredients:

- 1 (2-pound) boneless pork loin roast
- Sea salt
- Freshly ground black pepper
- 3 tablespoons olive oil
- 1½ cups heavy (whipping) cream
- 3 tablespoons grainy mustard, such as Pommery

Directions:

1. Preheat the oven to 375°F.
2. Season the pork roast all over with sea salt and pepper.
3. Place a large skillet over medium-high heat and add the olive oil.
4. Brown the roast on all sides in the skillet, about 6 minutes in total, and place the roast in a baking dish.
5. Roast until a meat thermometer inserted in the thickest part of the roast reads 155°F, about 1 hour.

6. When there is approximately 15 minutes of roasting time left, place a small saucepan over medium heat and add the heavy cream and mustard.
7. Stir the sauce until it simmers, then reduce the heat to low. Simmer the sauce until it is very rich and thick, about 5 minutes. Remove the pan from the heat and set aside.
8. Let the pork rest for 10 minutes before slicing and serve with the sauce.

Nutrition: Calories 368 Fat: 29g Protein: 25g Carbs: 2g Fiber: 0g Net Carbs: 2g Fat 70%/Protein 25%/Carbs 5%

151. Lamb Chops with Kalamata Tapenade

Preparation time: 15 minutes
Cooking time: 25 minutes
Servings: 4
Ingredients:
FOR THE TAPENADE

- 1 cup pitted Kalamata olives
- 2 tablespoons chopped fresh parsley
- 2 tablespoons extra-virgin olive oil
- 2 teaspoons minced garlic
- 2 teaspoons freshly squeezed lemon juice

FOR THE LAMB CHOPS

- 2 (1-pound) racks French-cut lamb chops (8 bones each)
- Sea salt
- Freshly ground black pepper
- 1 tablespoon olive oil

Directions:

1. Place the olives, parsley, olive oil, garlic, and lemon juice in a food processor and process until the mixture is puréed but still slightly chunky.
2. Transfer the tapenade to a container and store sealed in the refrigerator until needed.

TO MAKE THE LAMB CHOPS

3. Preheat the oven to 450°F.
4. Season the lamb racks with salt and pepper.
5. Place a large ovenproof skillet over medium-high heat and add the olive oil.
6. Pan sear the lamb racks on all sides until browned, about 5 minutes in total.
7. Arrange the racks upright in the skillet, with the bones interlaced, and roast them in the oven until they reach your desired doneness, about 20 minutes for medium-rare or until the internal temperature reaches 125°F.
8. Let the lamb rest for 10 minutes and then cut the lamb racks into chops. Arrange 4 chops per person on the plate and top with the Kalamata tapenade.

Nutrition: Calories: 348 Fat: 28g Protein: 21g Carbs: 2g Fiber: 1g Net Carbs: 1g Fat 72%/Protein 25%/Carbs 3%

152. Rosemary-Garlic Lamb Racks

Preparation time: 10 minutes, plus 1-hour marinating time
Cooking time: 25 minutes

Servings: 4
Ingredients:

- 4 tablespoons extra-virgin olive oil
- 2 tablespoons finely chopped fresh rosemary
- 2 teaspoons minced garlic
- Pinch sea salt
- 2 (1-pound) racks French-cut lamb chops (8 bones each)

Directions:

1. In a small bowl, whisk together the olive oil, rosemary, garlic, and salt.
2. Place the racks in a sealable freezer bag and pour the olive oil mixture into the bag. Massage the meat through the bag so it is coated with the marinade. Press the air out of the bag and seal it.
3. Marinate the lamb racks in the refrigerator for 1 to 2 hours.
4. Preheat the oven to 450°F.
5. Place a large ovenproof skillet over medium-high heat. Take the lamb racks out of the bag and sear them in the skillet on all sides, about 5 minutes in total.
6. Arrange the racks upright in the skillet, with the bones interlaced, and roast them in the oven until they reach your desired doneness, about 20 minutes for medium-rare or until the internal temperature reaches 125°F.
7. Let the lamb rest for 10 minutes and then cut the racks into chops.
8. Serve 4 chops per person.

Nutrition: Calories: 354 Fat: 30g Protein: 21g Carbs: 0g Fiber: 0g Net Carbs: 0g Fat 70%/Protein 30%/Carbs 0%

153. Lamb Leg with Sun-Dried Tomato Pesto

Preparation time: 15 minutes
Cooking time: 70 minutes
Servings: 8
Ingredients:
FOR THE PESTO

- 1 cup sun-dried tomatoes packed in oil, drained
- ¼ cup pine nuts
- 2 tablespoons extra-virgin olive oil
- 2 tablespoons chopped fresh basil
- 2 teaspoons minced garlic

FOR THE LAMB LEG

- 1 (2-pound) lamb leg
- Sea salt
- Freshly ground black pepper
- 2 tablespoons olive oil

Directions:
TO MAKE THE PESTO

1. Place the sun-dried tomatoes, pine nuts, olive oil, basil, and garlic in a blender or food processor; process until smooth.
2. Set aside until needed.

TO MAKE THE LAMB LEG

3. Preheat the oven to 400°F.
4. Season the lamb leg all over with salt and pepper.

5. Place a large ovenproof skillet over medium-high heat and add the olive oil.
6. Sear the lamb on all sides until nicely browned, about 6 minutes in total.
7. Spread the sun-dried tomato pesto all over the lamb and place the lamb on a baking sheet. Roast until the meat reaches your desired doneness, about 1 hour for medium.
8. Let the lamb rest for 10 minutes before slicing and serving.

Nutrition: Calories: 352 Fat: 29g Protein: 17g Carbs: 5g Fiber: 2g; Net Carbs: 3g Fat 74%/Protein 20%/Carbs 6%

154. Sirloin with Blue Cheese Compound Butter

Preparation time: 10 minutes, plus 1-hour chilling time
Cooking time: 12 minutes
Servings: 4
Ingredients:

- 6 tablespoons butter, at room temperature
- 4 ounces' blue cheese, such as Stilton or Roquefort
- 4 (5-ounce) beef sirloin steaks
- 1 tablespoon olive oil
- Sea salt
- Freshly ground black pepper

Directions:

1. Place the butter in a blender and pulse until the butter is whipped, about 2 minutes.
2. Add the cheese and pulse until just incorporated.
3. Spoon the butter mixture onto a sheet of plastic wrap and roll it into a log about 1½ inches in diameter by twisting both ends of the plastic wrap in opposite directions.
4. Refrigerate the butter until completely set, about 1 hour.
5. Slice the butter into ½-inch disks and set them on a plate in the refrigerator until you are ready to serve the steaks. Store leftover butter in the refrigerator for up to 1 week.
6. Preheat a barbecue to medium-high heat.
7. Let the steaks come to room temperature.
8. Rub the steaks all over with the olive oil and season them with salt and pepper.
9. Grill the steaks until they reach your desired doneness, about 6 minutes per side for medium.
10. If you do not have a barbecue, broil the steaks in a preheated oven for 7 minutes per side for medium.
11. Let the steaks rest for 10 minutes. Serve each topped with a disk of the compound butter.

Nutrition: Calories: 544 Fat: 44g Protein: 35g Carbs: 0g Fiber: 0g Net Carbs: 0g Fat 72%/Protein 28%/Carbs 0%

155. Garlic-Braised Short Rib

Preparation time: 10 minutes
Cooking time: 2 hours, 20 minutes
Servings: 4
Ingredients:

- 4 (4-ounce) beef short ribs
- Sea salt
- Freshly ground black pepper

- 1 tablespoon olive oil
- 2 teaspoons minced garlic
- ½ cup dry red wine
- 3 cups Rich Beef Stock (here)

Directions:

1. Preheat the oven to 325°F.
2. Season the beef ribs on all sides with salt and pepper.
3. Place a deep ovenproof skillet over medium-high heat and add the olive oil.
4. Sear the ribs on all sides until browned, about 6 minutes in total. Transfer the ribs to a plate.
5. Add the garlic to the skillet and sauté until translucent, about 3 minutes.
6. Whisk in the red wine to deglaze the pan. Be sure to scrape all the browned bits from the meat from the bottom of the pan. Simmer the wine until it is slightly reduced, about 2 minutes.
7. Add the beef stock, ribs, and any accumulated juices on the plate back to the skillet and bring the liquid to a boil.
8. Cover the skillet and place it in the oven to braise the ribs until the meat is fall-off-the-bone tender, about 2 hours.
9. Serve the ribs with a spoonful of the cooking liquid drizzled over each serving.

Nutrition: Calories: 481 Fat: 38g Protein: 29g Carbs: 5g Fiber: 3g Net Carbs: 2g Fat 70%/Protein 25%/Carbs 5%

156. Skirt Steak with Asian Peanut Sauce

Preparation Time: 15 minutes, plus 30 minutes to chill
Cooking Time: 15 minutes
Servings: 4
Ingredients:

- ⅓ cup light coconut milk
- 1 teaspoon curry powder
- 1 teaspoon coriander powder
- 1 teaspoon reduced-sodium soy sauce
- 1¼ pound skirt steak
- Cooking spray
- ½ cup Asian Peanut Sauce

Directions:

1. In a large bowl, whisk together the coconut milk, curry powder, coriander powder, and soy sauce. Add the steak and turn to coat. Cover the bowl and refrigerate for at least 30 minutes and no longer than 24 hours.
2. Preheat the barbecue or coat a grill pan with cooking spray and place the steak over medium-high heat. Grill the meat until it reaches an internal temperature of 145°F, about 3 minutes per side. Remove the steak from the grill and let it rest for 5 minutes. Slice the steak into 5-ounce pieces and serve each with 2 tablespoons of the Asian Peanut Sauce.
3. REFRIGERATE: Store the cooled steak in a reseal able container for up to 1 week. Reheat each piece in the microwave for 1 minute.

Nutrition: Calories: 361 Fat: 22g Saturated Fat: 7g Protein: 36g Total Carbs: 8g Fiber: 2g Sodium: 349mg

157. Tex-Mex Burgers

Preparation Time: 15 minutes
Cooking Time: 10 minutes
Servings: 4
Ingredients:

- 1-pound lean ground beef (90% or leaner)
- ¼ red onion, finely chopped
- ¼ green bell pepper, finely chopped
- ¼ cup chopped cilantro
- 2 garlic cloves, minced
- 1 teaspoon ground cumin
- 1 teaspoon smoked paprika
- ¼ teaspoon salt
- ⅛ teaspoon freshly ground black pepper
- ⅛ teaspoon allspice
- Cooking spray
- ½ cup Avocado Lime Mayonnaise

Directions:

1. In a medium bowl, combine the ground beef, onion, bell pepper, cilantro, garlic, cumin, paprika, salt, black pepper, and allspice. Using clean hands, form the mixture into 4 patties.
2. Coat a grill pan or sauté pan with the cooking spray and place it over medium heat. When the oil is shimmering, add the burgers and cook until a thermometer inserted into the center of a burger reads 155°F, about 5 minutes per side.
3. Top each burger with 2 tablespoons of the Avocado Lime Mayonnaise before eating.
4. REFRIGERATE: Store the cooled burgers and mayonnaise in separate resealable containers for up to 1 week. Reheat the burgers in the microwave for 1 to 2 minutes. They also can be reheated on the barbecue or in a grill pan for about 4 minutes per side. Top with the mayonnaise before eating.
5. FREEZE: Place the cooled burgers in a freezer-safe container for up to 2 months. Thaw in the refrigerator overnight and reheat in the microwave for 1 to 2 minutes. They can also be reheated on the grill or in a grill pan for about 4 minutes per side. The mayonnaise will not freeze well.

Nutrition: Calories: 267 Fat: 17g Saturated Fat: 5g Protein: 24g Total Carbs: 5g Fiber: 3g Sodium: 253mg

158. Beef Mushroom Meatballs

Preparation Time: 15 minutes
Cooking Time: 30 minutes
Servings: 24 meatballs
Ingredients:

- 1 tablespoon canola or safflower oil
- 1 (8-ounce) container Portobello mushrooms, finely chopped
- Cooking spray
- 1-pound lean ground beef (90% or higher)
- ¾ cup unseasoned bread crumbs
- ½ cup chopped fresh parsley

- 2 garlic cloves, minced
- 1 egg, beaten
- ¼ teaspoon salt
- ⅛ teaspoon freshly ground black pepper

Directions:

1. In a medium skillet over medium heat, heat the oil until it shimmers. Add the mushrooms and sauté until they soften, about 5 minutes. Set aside to slightly cool for 5 minutes.
2. Preheat the oven to 350ºF. Coat a mini muffin tin with the cooking spray.
3. In a large bowl, combine the mushrooms, beef, bread crumbs, parsley, garlic, egg, salt, and black pepper. Using clean hands, mix until well combined.
4. Form 1 heaping teaspoon of the beef mixture into a 2-inch ball. Place it into a muffin cup and continue forming meatballs.
5. Bake until the meatballs are golden brown, about 25 minutes. Let cool for 5 minutes, then use a teaspoon to transfer each meatball into a storage container.
6. REFRIGERATE: Store the cooled meatballs in a resealable container for up to 1 week. To reheat, microwave for 1 minute. The meatballs also can be reheated in a saucepan over medium heat along with the Speedy Tomato Sauce.
7. FREEZE: Store the cooled meatballs in a freezer-safe container for up to 2 months. Thaw in the refrigerator overnight and reheat in the microwave for 1 minute. The meatballs also can be reheated in a saucepan over medium heat along with the Speedy Tomato Sauce.

Nutrition: Calories: 232 Fat: 12g Saturated Fat: 4g Protein: 19g Total Carbs: 12g Fiber: 1g Sodium: 276mg

159. Lentil Beef Meatloaf

Preparation Time: 15 minutes
Cooking Time: 1 hour
Servings: 8
Ingredients:

- Cooking spray
- 1-pound lean ground beef (90% lean or higher)
- 1 (8-ounce) container mushrooms, finely chopped
- ½ onion, finely chopped
- 1 garlic clove, minced
- 1 (15-ounce) can low-sodium lentils, drained and rinsed
- ½ cup chopped fresh cilantro
- 1 large egg, beaten
- 1 cup whole-wheat panko bread crumbs
- ½ teaspoon salt
- ¼ teaspoon freshly ground black pepper
- ¾ cup Speedy Tomato Sauce

Directions:

1. Preheat the oven to 350ºF. Coat a 9-by-5-inch loaf pan with the cooking spray.

2. In a large bowl, combine the beef, mushrooms, onions, garlic, lentils, cilantro, egg, panko, salt, and black pepper. Mix until thoroughly combined.
3. Place the meat mixture into the loaf pan, making sure the top is even. Pour the tomato sauce over the top of the meatloaf.
4. Bake until a thermometer reads 155ºF when inserted into the center of the meatloaf, about 1 hour to 1 hour, 10 minutes.
5. . Let cool and slice into 8 equal portions.
6. REFRIGERATE: Store the cooled meatloaf slices in a resealable container for up to 1 week. Reheat in the microwave for 1 to 1½ minutes.
7. FREEZE: Store the cooled meatloaf slices in a freezer-safe container for up to 2 months. Thaw in the refrigerator overnight. Reheat in the microwave for 1 to 1½ minutes.

Nutrition: Calories: 210 Fat: 7g Saturated Fat: 3g Protein: 19g Total Carbs: 18g Fiber: 5g Sodium: 224mg

160. Mediterranean Stuffed Peppers

Preparation Time: 30 minutes, plus 30 minutes to chill
Cooking Time: 1 hour, 40 minutes
Servings: 8
Ingredients:

- 3 cups water
- 1 cup farro
- Cooking spray
- 1-pound lean ground beef (90% lean or higher)
- 1 cup reduced-sodium canned chickpeas, drained and rinsed
- 1 cup cherry tomatoes, quartered
- 1 bunch parsley, chopped
- ½ small yellow onion, chopped
- ⅓ cup crumbled feta cheese
- 3 tablespoons olive oil
- Juice of ½ lemon (about 1 tablespoon)
- ½ teaspoon salt
- ¼ teaspoon freshly ground black pepper
- 8 red, yellow, or green bell peppers

Directions:

1. In a medium pot over high heat, bring the water to a boil. Stir in the farro, then reduce the heat to medium-low and simmer until the water is absorbed and the grain is tender, about 30 minutes. Drain off any excess liquid. Let cool for about 10 minutes, then transfer to a container, cover, and refrigerate for at least 30 minutes.
2. Preheat the oven to 350ºF. Coat a 9-by-13-inch baking dish with the cooking spray.
3. In a large bowl, combine the beef, chickpeas, tomatoes, parsley, and onion and stir until well mixed. Add the chilled farro and feta cheese and stir to combine.
4. In a small bowl, whisk together the olive oil, lemon juice, salt, and black pepper. Pour this into the beef-farro mixture and stir to incorporate.

5. Slice the tops off the peppers. Using a paring knife, remove the membranes and seeds from inside each pepper. Spoon ¾ cup of the beef mixture into each pepper and arrange the peppers in the baking dish, leaving about 2 inches between them. Cover the dish with aluminum foil.

6. Bake for 50 minutes. Then remove the foil and continue baking for another 20 minutes.

7. REFRIGERATE: Store the cooled peppers in a resealable container for up to 1 week. Reheat one pepper in the microwave for 1 to 2 minutes. To reheat more evenly, slice the pepper in quarters.

8. FREEZE: Store the cooled peppers in a freezer-safe container for up to 2 months. Thaw in the refrigerator overnight. Reheat one pepper in the microwave for 1 to 2 minutes. To reheat more evenly, slice the pepper in quarters.

Nutrition: Calories: 320 Fat: 14g Saturated Fat: 4g Protein: 19g Total Carbs: 30g Fiber: 7g Sodium: 291mg

161. Classic Mini Meatloaf

Preparation Time: 10 minutes
Cooking Time: 25 minutes
Servings: 6
Ingredients:

- 1 pound 80/20 ground beef
- ¼ medium yellow onion, peeled and diced
- ½ medium green bell pepper, seeded and diced
- 1 large egg
- 3 tablespoons blanched finely ground almond flour
- 1 tablespoon Worcestershire sauce
- ½ teaspoon garlic powder
- 1 teaspoon dried parsley
- 2 tablespoons tomato paste
- ¼ cup water
- 1 tablespoon powdered erythritol

Directions:

1. In a large bowl, combine ground beef, onion, pepper, egg, and almond flour. Pour in the Worcestershire sauce and add the garlic powder and parsley to the bowl. Mix until fully combined.

2. Divide the mixture into two and place into two (4") loaf baking pans.

3. In a small bowl, mix the tomato paste, water, and erythritol. Spoon half the mixture over each loaf.

4. Working in batches if necessary, place loaf pans into the air fryer basket.

5. Adjust the temperature to 350°F and set the timer for 25 minutes or until internal temperature is 180°F.

6. Serve warm.

Nutrition: Calories: 170 Protein: 14.9 G Fiber: 0.9 G Net Carbohydrates: 2.6 G Sugar Alcohol: 1.5 G Fat: 9.4 G Sodium: 85 Mg Carbohydrates: 5.0 G Sugar: 1.5 G

162. Chorizo and Beef Burger

Preparation Time: 10 minutes
Cooking Time: 15 minutes
Servings: 4
Ingredients:

- ¾ pound 80/20 ground beef
- ¼ pound Mexican-style ground chorizo
- ¼ cup chopped onion
- 5 slices pickled jalapeños, chopped
- 2 teaspoons chili powder
- 1 teaspoon minced garlic
- ¼ teaspoon cumin

Directions:

1. In a large bowl, mix all ingredients. Divide the mixture into four sections and form them into burger patties.

2. Place burger patties into the air fryer basket, working in batches if necessary.

3. Adjust the temperature to 375°F and set the timer for 15 minutes.

4. Flip the patties halfway through the cooking time. Serve warm.

Nutrition: Calories: 291 Protein: 21.6 G Fiber: 0.9 G Net Carbohydrates: 3.8 G Fat: 18.3 G Sodium: 474 Mg Carbohydrates: 4.7 G Sugar: 2.5 G

163. Crispy Brats

Preparation Time: 5 minutes
Cooking Time: 15 minutes
Servings: 4
Ingredients:

- 4 (3-ounce) beef bratwursts

Directions:

1. Place brats into the air fryer basket.

2. Adjust the temperature to 375°F and set the timer for 15 minutes.

3. Serve warm.

Nutrition: Calories: 286 Protein: 11.8 G Fiber: 0.0 G Fat: 24.8 G Sodium: 50 Mg Carbohydrates: 0.0 G Sugar: 0.0 G

164. Taco-Stuffed Peppers

Preparation Time: 15 minutes
Cooking Time: 15 minutes
Servings: 4
Ingredients:

- 1 pound 80/20 ground beef
- 1 tablespoon chili powder
- 2 teaspoons cumin
- 1 teaspoon garlic powder
- 1 teaspoon salt
- ¼ teaspoon ground black pepper
- 1 (10-ounce) can diced tomatoes and green chiles, drained
- 4 medium green bell peppers
- 1 cup shredded Monterey jack cheese, divided

Directions:

1. In a medium skillet over medium heat, brown the ground beef about 7–10 minutes. When no pink remains, drain the fat from the skillet.

2. Return the skillet to the stovetop and add chili powder, cumin, garlic powder, salt, and black pepper. Add drained can of diced tomatoes and chiles to the skillet. Continue cooking 3–5 minutes.

3. While the mixture is cooking, cut each bell pepper in half. Remove the seeds and white membrane.

Spoon the cooked mixture evenly into each bell pepper and top with a ¼ cup cheese. Place stuffed peppers into the air fryer basket.

4. Adjust the temperature to 350°F and set the timer for 15 minutes.
5. When done, peppers will be fork tender and cheese will be browned and bubbling. Serve warm.

Nutrition: Calories: 346 Protein: 27.8 G Fiber: 3.5 G Net Carbohydrates: 7.2 G Fat: 19.1 G Sodium: 991 Mg Carbohydrates: 10.7 G Sugar: 4.9 G

165. **Italian Stuffed Bell Peppers**

Preparation Time: 15 minutes
Cooking Time: 15 minutes
Servings: 4
Ingredients:

- 1-pound ground pork Italian sausage
- ½ teaspoon garlic powder
- ½ teaspoon dried parsley
- 1 medium Roma tomato, diced
- ¼ cup chopped onion
- 4 medium green bell peppers
- 1 cup shredded mozzarella cheese, divided

Ingredients:

1. In a medium skillet over medium heat, brown the ground sausage about 7–10 minutes or until no pink remains. Drain the fat from the skillet.
2. Return the skillet to the stovetop and add garlic powder, parsley, tomato, and onion. Continue cooking 3–5 minutes.
3. Slice peppers in half and remove the seeds and white membrane.
4. Remove the meat mixture from the stovetop and spoon evenly into pepper halves. Top with mozzarella. Place pepper halves into the air fryer basket.
5. Adjust the temperature to 350°F and set the timer for 15 minutes.
6. When done, peppers will be fork tender and cheese will be golden. Serve warm.

Nutrition: Calories: 358 Protein: 21.1 G Fiber: 2.6 G Net Carbohydrates: 8.7 G Fat: 24.1 G Sodium: 1,029 Mg Carbohydrates: 11.3 G Sugar: 4.8 G

166. **Bacon Cheeseburger Casserole**

Preparation Time: 15 minutes
Cooking Time: 20 minutes
Servings: 4
Ingredients:

- 1 pound 80/20 ground beef
- ¼ medium white onion, peeled and chopped
- 1 cup shredded Cheddar cheese, divided
- 1 large egg
- 4 slices sugar-free bacon, cooked and crumbled
- 2 pickle spears, chopped

Directions:

1. Brown the ground beef in a medium skillet over medium heat about 7–10 minutes. When no pink

remains, drain the fat. Remove from heat and add ground beef to large mixing bowl.

2. Add onion, ½ cup Cheddar, and egg to bowl. Mix ingredients well and add crumbled bacon.
3. Pour the mixture into a 4-cup round baking dish and top with remaining Cheddar. Place into the air fryer basket.
4. Adjust the temperature to 375°F and set the timer for 20 minutes.
5. Casserole will be golden on top and firm in the middle when fully cooked. Serve immediately with chopped pickles on top.

Nutrition: Calories: 369 Protein: 31.0 G Fiber: 0.2 G Net Carbohydrates: 1.0 G Fat: 22.6 G Sodium: 454 Mg Carbohydrates: 1.2 G Sugar: 0.5 G

167. **Pulled Pork**

Preparation Time: 10 minutes
Cooking Time: 2½ hours
Servings: 8
Ingredients:

- 2 tablespoons chili powder
- 1 teaspoon garlic powder
- ½ teaspoon onion powder
- ½ teaspoon ground black pepper
- ½ teaspoon cumin

Directions:

1. 1 (4-pound) pork shoulder
2. In a small bowl, mix chili powder, garlic powder, onion powder, pepper, and cumin. Rub the spice mixture over the pork shoulder, patting it into the skin. Place pork shoulder into the air fryer basket.
3. Adjust the temperature to 350°F and set the timer for 150 minutes.
4. Pork skin will be crispy and meat easily shredded with two forks when done. The internal temperature should be at least 145°F.

Nutrition: Calories: 537 Protein: 42.6 G Fiber: 0.8 G Net Carbohydrates: 0.7 G Fat: 35.5 G Sodium: 180 Mg Carbohydrates: 1.5 G Sugar: 0.2 G

168. **Baby Back Ribs**

Preparation Time: 5 minutes
Cooking Time: 25 minutes
Servings: 4
Ingredients:

- 2 pounds' baby back ribs
- 2 teaspoons chili powder
- 1 teaspoon paprika
- ½ teaspoon onion powder
- ½ teaspoon garlic powder
- ¼ teaspoon ground cayenne pepper
- ½ cup low-carb, sugar-free barbecue sauce

Directions:

1. Rub ribs with all ingredients except barbecue sauce. Place into the air fryer basket.
2. Adjust the temperature to 400°F and set the timer for 25 minutes.

3. When done, ribs will be dark and charred with an internal temperature of at least 190°F. Brush ribs with barbecue sauce and serve warm.

Nutrition: Calories: 650 Protein: 40.1 G Fiber: 0.8 G Net Carbohydrates: 2.8 G Fat: 51.5 G Sodium: 332 Mg Carbohydrates: 3.6 G Sugar: 0.2 G

169. **Bacon-Wrapped Hot Dog**

Preparation Time: 5 minutes
Cooking Time: 10 minutes
Servings: 4
Ingredients:

- 4 beef hot dogs
- 4 slices sugar-free bacon

Directions:

1. Wrap each hot dog with slice of bacon and secure with toothpick. Place into the air fryer basket.
2. Adjust the temperature to 370°F and set the timer for 10 minutes.
3. Flip each hot dog halfway through the cooking time. When fully cooked, bacon will be crispy. Serve warm.

Nutrition: Calories: 197 Protein: 9.2 G Fiber: 0.0 G Net Carbohydrates: 1.3 G Fat: 15.0 G Sodium: 571 Mg Carbohydrates: 1.3 G Sugar: 0.6 G

170. **Easy Juicy Pork Chops**

Preparation Time: 5 minutes
Cooking Time: 15 minutes
Servings: 2
Ingredients:

- 1 teaspoon chili powder
- ½ teaspoon garlic powder
- ½ teaspoon cumin
- ¼ teaspoon ground black pepper
- ¼ teaspoon dried oregano
- 2 (4-ounce) boneless pork chops
- 2 tablespoons unsalted butter, divided

Directions:

1. In a small bowl, mix chili powder, garlic powder, cumin, pepper, and oregano. Rub dry rub onto pork chops. Place pork chops into the air fryer basket.
2. Adjust the temperature to 400°F and set the timer for 15 minutes.
3. The internal temperature should be at least 145°F when fully cooked. Serve warm, each topped with 1 tablespoon butter.

Nutrition: Calories: 313 Protein: 24.4 G Fiber: 0.7 G Net Carbohydrates: 1.1 G Fat: 22.6 G Sodium: 117 Mg Carbohydrates: 1.8 G Sugar: 0.1 G

171. **Pork Roast**

Preparation Time: 10 minutes
Cooking Time: 3 hours
Servings: 2
Ingredients:

- Coconut oil (1 T)
- Water (2 c)
- Portobello mushrooms (5 sliced thin)
- Garlic (2 cloves smashed)
- Onion (.5 chopped)
- Celery (1 rib)
- Pepper (.5 tsp.)
- Pork roast (1 lb.)

Directions:

1. Start by adding the garlic onion and celery to the Instant Pot cooker pot before adding in the water and then the roast, before seasoning as desired.
2. Place the Instant Pot cooker pot into the Instant Pot cooker and seal the lid. Choose the high-pressure option and set the time for 60 minutes.
3. Once the timer goes off, choose the instant pressure release option
4. Set the roast aside and place the vegetables and resulting broth into a blender and blend well.
5. Place the roast back in the Instant Pot cooker, seal the cooker and allow it to cook for 2 hours under high pressure, this will help to render the fat and ensure the edges are crisp.
6. When the timer goes off, use the instant pressure release option and transfer the roast to a serving dish.
7. Turn the Instant Pot cooker to the sauté setting before adding in the coconut oil. Once it is heated, add in the mushrooms and allow them to cook for 5 minutes. Add in the gravy from the blender and let it reduce until desired thickness is achieved.
8. Top roast with gravy prior to serving.

Nutrition: Protein: 23.8 grams Carbs: 13.2 grams Fiber: 9 grams Sugar: 2.2 grams Fats: 3.5 grams Calories: 360

172. **Pork Curry**

Preparation Time: 10 minutes
Cooking Time: 20 minutes
Servings: 2
Ingredients:

- Carrots (2 sliced)
- Turmeric (.25 tsp.)
- Garam masala (1.5 T)
- Diced tomatoes (4 oz.)
- Zucchini (.25 diced)
- Ghee (1 T)
- Black pepper (1 pinch)
- Coconut milk (.5 c)
- Onion (.5 diced)
- Lime juice (.5 limes)
- Ginger (1 inch grated)
- Garlic (2 cloves minced)
- Pork (1 lb.)

Directions:

1. In a sealable container, place the meat before adding in the coconut milk, garlic, lime juice and ginger and mixing thoroughly. Allow the meat to marinate overnight for best results.
2. Place the onions, carrots, garam masala, ghee, tomatoes and meat together in the Instant Pot cooker pot and combine thoroughly.
3. Place the Instant Pot cooker pot into the Instant Pot cooker and seal the lid. Choose the high-pressure option and set the time for 20 minutes.

4. Once the timer goes off, select the natural pressure release option and allow the pot to sit for 10 minutes
5. After opening the lid, switch the Instant Pot cooker to sauté before adding in the zucchini and letting it simmer for 5 minutes.
6. Serve hot over shirataki rice.

Nutrition: Protein: 38 grams Carbs: 29 grams Fiber: 23 grams Sugar: 3.5 grams Fats: 33 grams Calories: 520

173. Carnitas

Preparation Time: 30 minutes
Cooking Time: 50 minutes
Servings: 2
Ingredients:

- Bay leaves (1)
- Garlic (1 clove slivered)
- Oregano (.25 tsp)
- Garlic powder (.25 tsp)
- Adobo seasoning (.25 tsp.)
- Low-sodium vegetable broth (.25 c)
- Cumin (.5 tsp.)
- Roast (1 lb.)
- Chipotle pepper with adobo sauce (1)

Directions:

1. Set your Instant Pot cooker to sauté.
2. Season the pork as desired before adding it to the Instant Pot cooker and cooking each side for about 5 minutes. Remove the pork from the pot and set aside to cool.
3. With the help of a sharp knife, make a 1-in. incision in the pork that is deep enough to accept the garlic slivers.
4. Add additional seasonings to the pork as desired, rub the mixture into the meat.
5. Add the broth, bay leaf and the chipotle pepper to the Instant Pot before placing it in the Instant Pot cooker pot and sealing the lid of the cooker. Choose the high-pressure option and set the time for 50 minutes.
6. Once the timer goes off, select the instant pressure release option and remove the lid. Remove the pork and shred using a pair of forks.
7. Return the pork to the Instant Pot cooker and allow it to soak up any remaining juices, taking care to remove bay before doing so.

Nutrition: Protein: 20 grams Carbs: 12.2 grams Fiber: 11.9 grams Sugar: 11.2 grams Fats: 7.5 grams Calories: 320

174. Cherry Apple Pork

Preparation Time: 5 minutes
Cooking Time: 40 minutes
Servings: 2
Ingredients:

- Apple (1 small, diced)
- Cherries (.3 c pitted)
- Onion (3 T diced)
- Celery (3 T diced)
- Apple juice (.25 c)
- Black pepper

- Pork loin (.75 lb.)
- Water (.25 c)

Direction:

1. Add all of the ingredients to the Instant Pot cooker and mix thoroughly.
2. Seal the lid of the cooker, choose the poultry setting and set the time for 5 minutes.
3. Once the timer goes off, select the quick pressure release option and remove the lid as soon as the pressure has normalized.
4. Serve warm.

Nutrition: Protein: 12 grams Carbs: 22.9 grams Fiber: 19 grams Sugar: 11.2 grams Fats: 28 grams Calories: 453

175. Pork Chops and Cabbage

Preparation Time: 10 minutes
Cooking Time: 15 minutes
Servings: 2
Ingredients:

- Pork chops (2)
- Fennel seeds (.5 tsp.)
- Black pepper (as desired)
- Cabbage (1 small head)
- Coconut oil (1.5 tsp.)
- Beef stock (.3 c)
- Almond flour (1 tsp.)

Directions:

1. Preheat cooker on sauté.
2. Sprinkle the chops with pepper, fennel, and salt.
3. Slice the cabbage into ¾ inch slices, set aside.
4. In preheated cooker, add oil and brown the chops on one side.
5. Remove the chops and add the cabbage.
6. Place the chops browned side up on the cabbage. Pour in the stock.
7. Cover and seal with lid.
8. Cook 8 minutes on high pressure.
9. Once finished, release the pressure. Remove the meat and cabbage and tent with foil.
10. Allow the juices to boil. Stir in the flour. Pour the sauce over the meat and cabbage and serve. Once the timer goes off, select the natural pressure release option and remove the lid as soon as the pressure has normalized.
11. Serve warm.

Nutrition: Protein: 31 grams Carbs: 35 grams Fiber: 26 grams Sugar: 11.2 grams Fats: 18.2 grams Calories: 412

176. Root Beer Pork

Preparation Time: 15 minutes
Cooking Time: 35 minutes
Servings: 2
Ingredients:

- Pork roast (1 lb.)
- Black pepper (as desired)
- Onion (.6 c sliced)
- Root beet (.3 c)
- Ketchup (2 T)
- Almond flour (1.5 tsp)

- Lemon juice (.25 tsp) / Worcestershire sauce (1.5 tsp)
- Tomato paste (1 T) / Honey (1.5 tsp)

Directions:

1. Season roast with pepper and garlic salt, and put in the pot.
2. Mix the rest of the ingredients together and pour on the roast.
3. Lock and seal the lid.
4. Set to meat/stew for 35 minutes. Carefully release pressure
5. Take out onions and roast.
6. Discard the onions and shred the pork.
7. Stir the pork back into the pot.

Nutrition: Protein: 19.7grams Carbs: 26.2 grams Fiber: 21.5 grams Sugar: 0 grams Fats: 17.2 grams Calories: 323

177. Maple Glazed Pork

Preparation Time: 10 minutes
Cooking Time: 15 minutes
Servings: 2
Ingredients:

- Maple syrup (.25 c)
- Honey (.25 c)
- Cinnamon (1 tsp)
- Brown sugar (.25 c)
- Orange juice (2 T)
- Nutmeg (1 tsp)
- Bone in ham (1 small)

Directions:

1. Combine everything except for the ham in a saucepan on medium heat; mix well.
2. Put the ham in the cooker. Cook 15 minutes, then use quick release.
3. Set the ham in the baking dish. Pour glaze over ham.
4. Place the ham under a broiler to caramelize the sugars and form a slight char.

Nutrition: Protein: 23.8 grams Carbs: 37.5 grams Fiber: 32.8 grams Sugar: 18.2 grams Fats: 42 grams Calories: 540

178. Air Fryer Roast Beef

Preparation Time: 5 minutes
Cooking Time: 45 minutes
Servings: 3
Ingredients:

- 3-1/2 lbs. beef roast
- 2 tbsps. olive oil
- 1 tbsp. rosemary
- 1/2 tbsp. garlic powder
- 1/2 tsp fresh ground rugged black pepper

Directions:

1. Adjust the temperature of the air fryer to 360°F
2. Mix herbs and oil on a plate. Roll the roast in the blend on the plate to ensure that the entire surface of the beef is covered.
3. Set the beef in the air fryer basket. Establish the timer for 45 mins for tool-rare beef, 51 mins for the tool. Examine the beef with a meat thermostat to see if it is done to your liking.

4. Cook for extra 6-minute periods if you like it cooked a lot more. Keep in mind that the roast will undoubtedly remain to prepare while it is relaxing.
5. Eliminate the roast from the air fryer and put on a plate, cover with lightweight aluminum foil. Allow it to rest for 10 minutes before serving.

Nutrition: Calories: 666 kcal; Carbs: 0.3g; Fat: 54g; Proteins: 43g

179. Air Fryer Bacon

Preparation Time: 5 minutes
Cooking Time: 10 minutes
Servings: 4
Ingredients:

- 11 slices bacon

Directions:

1. Divide the bacon in half, and place the first half in the air fryer.
2. Set the temperature at 401 degrees F, and set the timer to 11 mins.
3. Check it halfway through to see if anything needs to be rearranged.
4. Cook remainder of the time. Serve.

Nutrition: Calories: 91 kcal Carbs: 0g Protein: 2g Fat: 8g

180. Air Fryer Beef Empanadas

Preparation Time: 10 minutes
Cooking Time: 20 minutes
Servings: 3
Ingredients:

- 8 Goya empanada discs, defrosted
- 1 cup picadillo
- 1 egg white, blended
- 1 tsp. water
- Cooking spray

Directions:

1. Set air fryer at 325 degrees F.
2. Apply a cooking spray to the basket.
3. Place 2 tbsps. of picadillo to each disc space. Fold in half and secure using a fork. Do the same for all the dough.
4. Mix water and egg whites. Sprinkle to empanadas top.
5. Set 3 of them in your air fryer and allow to bake for minutes. Set aside and do the same for the remaining empanadas.

Nutrition: Calories:183 kcal Carbs: 22g Protein:11 g Fat:5g

181. Pork Rind

Preparation Time: 10 minutes
Cooking Time: 1 hr
Servings: 4
Ingredients:

- 1kg pork rinds
- Salt
- 1/2 tsp black pepper coffee

Direction:

1. Preheat the air fryer. Set the time of 5 minutes and the temperature to 2000C.
2. Cut the bacon into cubes - 1 finger wide.
3. Season with salt and a pinch of pepper.

4. Place in the basket of the air fryer. Set the time of 45 minutes and press the power button.
5. Shake the basket every 10 minutes so that the pork rinds stay golden brown equally.
6. Once they are ready, drain a little on the paper towel, so they stay dry. Transfer to a plate and serve.

Nutrition: Calories: 172 kcal Fat: 10.02g Carbs: 0g Protein: 19.62g

182. Pork Fillets with Serrano Ham

Preparation Time: 10 minutes
Cooking Time: 20 minutes
Servings: 4
Ingredients:
- 400g of very thin sliced pork fillets
- 2 boiled and chopped eggs
- 100g chopped Serrano ham
- 1 beaten egg
- Breadcrumbs

Direction:
1. Make a roll with the pork fillets. Introduce half-cooked egg and Serrano ham. So that the roll does not lose its shape, fasten with a string or chopsticks.
2. Pass the rolls through the beaten egg and then through the breadcrumbs until it forms a good layer.
3. Adjust the temperature of the air fryer for a few minutes at 180° C.
4. Insert the rolls in the basket and set the timer for about 8 minutes at 180° C.
5. Serve.

Nutrition: Calories: 424 kcal Fat: 15.15g Carbs: 37.47g Protein: 31.84g

183. Pork on A Blanket

Preparation Time: 5 minutes
Cooking Time: 10 minutes
Servings: 4
Ingredients:
- 1/2 puff defrosted pastry sheet
- 16 thick smoked sausages
- 15 ml of milk

Directions:
1. Adjust the temperature of the air fryer to 200°C and set the timer to 5 minutes.
2. Cut the puff pastry into 64 x 38 mm strips.
3. Place a cocktail sausage at the end of the puff pastry and roll around the sausage, sealing the dough with some water.
4. Brush the top of the sausages wrapped in milk and place them in the preheated air fryer.
5. Cook at 200°C for 10 minutes or until golden brown.

Nutrition: Calories: 242 kcal Fat: 14g Carbs: 0g Protein: 27g

184. Provencal Ribs

Preparation Time: 10 minutes
Cooking Time: 20 minutes
Servings: 4

Ingredients:
- 500g of pork ribs
- Provencal herbs
- Salt
- Ground pepper
- Oil

Direction:
1. Put the ribs in a bowl and add some oil, Provencal herbs, salt, and ground pepper.
2. Stir well and leave in the fridge for at least 1 hour.
3. Put the ribs in the basket of the air fryer and select 2000C for 20 minutes.
4. From time to time, shake the basket and remove the ribs.

Nutrition: Calories: 296 kcal Fat: 22.63g Carbs: 0g Protein: 21.71g

185. Marinated Loin Potatoes

Preparation Time: 20 minutes
Cooking Time: 1 hr
Servings: 4
Ingredients:
- 2 medium potatoes
- 4 fillets of marinated loin
- A little extra virgin olive oil
- Salt

Directions:
1. Peel the potatoes and cut. Cut with match-sized mandolin, potatoes with a cane but very thin.
2. Wash and immerse in water 30 minutes.
3. Drain and dry well.
4. Add a little oil and stir so that the oil permeates well in all the potatoes.
5. Go to the basket of the air fryer and distribute well.
6. Cook at 1600C for 10 minutes.
7. Take out the basket, shake so that the potatoes take off. Let the potato tender. If it is not, leave 5 more minutes.
8. Place the steaks on top of the potatoes.
9. Select, 10 minutes, and 1800C for 5 minutes again.

Nutrition: Calories: 136 kcal Fat: 5.1g Carbs: 1.9g Protein: 20.7g

186. Pork Tenderloin

Preparation Time: 10 minutes
Cooking Time: 30 minutes
Servings: 6
Ingredients:
- 1-1/2 lbs. pork tenderloin

Directions:
1. Adjust the temperature of the Air Fryer to 3700F.
2. Lay the pork in the Air Fryer basket.
3. Cook at 4000F for about 30 minutes, turning halfway through cooking time for a proper cook.
4. Serve.

Nutrition: Calories: 419 kcal; Fat: 3.5g; Carbs: 0g; Proteins: 26g

187. Roast Pork

Preparation Time: 10 minutes
Cooking Time: 30 minutes

Servings: 6
Ingredients:

- 2 lbs. pork loin
- 1 Tbsp. olive oil
- 1 tsp. salt

Directions:

1. Adjust the temperature of the Air Fryer to 360⁰F.
2. Apply the oil on the pork.
3. Add salt.
4. Cook the pork in the Air Fryer for about 50 minutes. Shake the food halfway through the cooking
5. Remove the meal from Air Fryer and allow it to cool.
6. Serve

Nutrition: Calories: 150 kcal Fat: 6g; Carbs: 0g; Protein: 23.1g

188. Pork Loin

Preparation Time: 10 minutes
Cooking Time: 20 minutes
Servings: 6
Ingredients:

- 1/2 lb. pork tenderloin patted dry
- Non-stick cooking spray
- 2 tbsps. garlic scape pesto
- Salt
- Pepper

Directions:

1. Adjust the temperature of the Air Fryer to 375⁰F.
2. Rub all sides of the tenderloin with the non-stick cooking spray
3. Add pepper, garlic scape pesto, and salt.
4. Sprinkle the Air Fryer basket with cooking spray.
5. Place the tenderloin on the Air Fryer.
6. Cook the meal at 400°F for 10 minutes.
7. Flip over to the other side and cook for another 10 minutes on the first side.
8. Remove the food from the air fryer.
9. Serve

Nutrition: Calories: 379 kcal Protein: 8.4g; Fat: 2.2g; Carbs: 0g

189. Pork Bondiola Chop

Preparation Time: 5 minutes
Cooking Time: 20 minutes
Servings: 4
Ingredients:

- 1kg bondiola in pieces
- Breadcrumbs
- 2 beaten eggs
- Seasoning to taste

Directions:

1. Cut the bondiola into small pieces.
2. Add seasonings to taste.
3. Pour the beaten eggs on the seasoned bondiola.
4. Add the breadcrumbs.
5. Cook in the air fryer for 20 minutes while turning the food halfway.
6. Serve

Nutrition: Calories: 265 kcal; Fat: 20.36g; Carbs: 0g; Protein: 19.14g;

190. Air Fryer Steak

Preparation Time: 5 minutes
Cooking Time: 10 minutes
Servings: 2
Ingredients:

- 1 Ribeye Steak or New York City Strip Steak
- Salt and Pepper
- Garlic Powder
- Paprika
- Butter

Directions:

1. Place the meat to sit in a bowl at room temperature level.
2. Spray the olive oil onto both sides of the steak.
3. Add salt and pepper to season.
4. Add the garlic powder and paprika to the mixture.
5. Adjust the temperature of the air fryer to 400F.
6. Place steak in the air fryer and cook for 12 minutes flipping it halfway through.
7. Lead it with butter when ready, then serve.

Nutrition: Calories: 301 kcal Fat: 23g Carbs: 0g Protein: 23g

191. Roast Beef

Preparation Time: 5 minutes
Cooking Time: 45 minutes
Servings: 4
Ingredients:

- 1 kg Beef Joint
- 1 tbsp. Extra Virgin Oliver Oil
- Salt
- Pepper

Directions:

1. Rub the beef with extra virgin olive oil.
2. Season with pepper and salt.
3. Then place the seasoned beef onto the air fryer oven rotisserie and put in place.
4. Adjust the timer to 45 minutes and the temperature to 380⁰F. Ensure the beef is rotating.
5. After the 45 minutes, check the readiness then slice the roast beef to pieces.
6. Serve

Nutrition: Calories: 666kcal Protein:43g Fat:54g

192. Traditional Beef Stew

Preparation Time: 15 minutes
Cooking Time: 35 minutes
Servings: 2
Ingredients:

- 1lb diced stewing steak
- 1lb chopped vegetables
- 1 cup low sodium beef broth
- 1tbsp black pepper

Directions:

1. Mix all the ingredients in your Instant Pot.
2. Cook on Stew for 35 minutes.
3. Release the pressure naturally.

Nutrition: Calories: 300 Carbs: 6 Sugar: 1 Fat: 9 Protein: 43 GL: 2

193. Steak and Kidney Stew

Preparation Time: 15 minutes
Cooking time: 35 minutes
Servings: 2
Ingredients:

- 1lb diced stewing steak
- 0.5lb diced kidneys
- 1lb chopped vegetables
- 1 cup low sodium beef broth
- 0.5 cup low carb beer

Directions:

1. Mix all the ingredients in your Instant Pot.
2. Cook on Stew for 35 minutes.
3. Release the pressure naturally.

Nutrition: Calories: 380 Carbs: 10 Sugar: 3 Fat: 12 Protein: 48 GL: 4

194. Slow Cooked Lamb

Preparation Time: 15 minutes
Cooking time: 35 minutes
Servings: 2
Ingredients:

- 1lb diced lean lamb
- 1 quartered onion
- 2 chopped carrots
- 1 cup low sodium broth
- 0.5 cup mint sauce

Directions:

1. Place the lamb in your Instant Pot.
2. Place the onion and carrots around it.
3. Pour the sauce and broth over it.
4. Cook on Stew for 35 minutes.
5. Release the pressure naturally.

Nutrition: Calories: 400 Carbs: 14 Sugar: 4 Fat: 20 Protein: 37 GL: 6

195. Honey Mustard Pork

Preparation Time: 15 minutes
Cooking time: 60 minutes
Servings: 2
Ingredients:

- 1.5lb rolled, trimmed pork joint
- 1 cup honey mustard sauce, low carb
- salt and pepper

Directions:

1. Mix all the ingredients in your Instant Pot.
2. Cook on Stew for 60 minutes.
3. Release the pressure naturally.

Nutrition: Calories: 290 Carbs: 9 Sugar: 8 Fat: 17 Protein: 39 GL: 4

196. Shredded Beef

Preparation Time: 15 minutes
Cooking time: 35 minutes
Servings: 2
Ingredients:

- 1.5lb lean steak
- 1 cup low sodium gravy
- 2tbsp mixed spices

Directions:

1. Mix all the ingredients in your Instant Pot.
2. Cook on Stew for 35 minutes.
3. Release the pressure naturally.
4. Shred the beef.

Nutrition: Calories: 200 Carbs: 2 Sugar: 0 Fat: 5 Protein: 48 GL: 1

197. Italian Sausage Casserole

Preparation Time: 15 minutes
Cooking time: 5 minutes
Servings: 2
Ingredients:

- 1lb chopped cooked sausages
- 1lb chopped Mediterranean vegetables
- 1 cup low sodium broth
- 1tbsp mixed herbs

Directions:

1. Mix all the ingredients in your Instant Pot.
2. Cook on Stew for 5 minutes.
3. Release the pressure naturally.

Nutrition: Calories: 320 Carbs: 8 Sugar: 2 Fat: 18 Protein: 41 GL: 4

FISH AND SEAFOOD RECIPES

198. Baked Salmon with Garlic Parmesan Topping

Preparation time: 5 minutes,
Cooking time: 20 minutes,
Servings: 4
Ingredients:

- 1 lb. wild caught salmon filets
- 2 tbsp. margarine
- What you'll need from store cupboard:
- ¼ cup reduced fat parmesan cheese, grated
- ¼ cup light mayonnaise
- 2-3 cloves garlic, diced
- 2 tbsp. parsley
- Salt and pepper

Directions:

1. Heat oven to 350 and line a baking pan with parchment paper.
2. Place salmon on pan and season with salt and pepper.
3. In a medium skillet, over medium heat, melt butter. Add garlic and cook, stirring 1 minute.
4. Reduce heat to low and add remaining Ingredients. Stir until everything is melted and combined.
5. Spread evenly over salmon and bake 15 minutes for thawed fish or 20 for frozen. Salmon is done when it flakes easily with a fork. Serve.

Nutrition: Calories 408 Total Carbs 4g Protein 41g Fat 24g Sugar 1g Fiber 0g

199. Blackened Shrimp

Preparation time: 5 minutes
Cooking time: 5 minutes
Servings: 4
Ingredients:

- 1 ½ lbs. shrimp, peel & devein
- 4 lime wedges
- 4 tbsp. cilantro, chopped
- What you'll need from store cupboard:
- 4 cloves garlic, diced
- 1 tbsp. chili powder
- 1 tbsp. paprika
- 1 tbsp. olive oil
- 2 tsp Splenda brown sugar
- 1 tsp cumin
- 1 tsp oregano
- 1 tsp garlic powder
- 1 tsp salt
- ½ tsp pepper

Directions:

1. In a small bowl combine seasonings and Splenda brown sugar.
2. Heat oil in a skillet over med-high heat. Add shrimp, in a single layer, and cook 1-2 minutes per side.

3. Add seasonings, and cook, stirring, 30 seconds. Serve garnished with cilantro and a lime wedge.

Nutrition: Calories 252 Total Carbs 7g Net Carbs 6g Protein 39g Fat 7g Sugar 2g Fiber 1g

200. Cajun Catfish

Preparation time: 5 minutes
Cooking time: 15 minutes
Servings: 4
Ingredients:

- 4 (8 oz.) catfish fillets
- What you'll need from store cupboard:
- 2 tbsp. olive oil
- 2 tsp garlic salt
- 2 tsp thyme
- 2 tsp paprika
- ½ tsp cayenne pepper
- ½ tsp red hot sauce
- ¼ tsp black pepper
- Nonstick cooking spray

Directions:

1. Heat oven to 450 degrees. Spray a 9x13-inch baking dish with cooking spray.
2. In a small bowl whisk together everything but catfish. Brush both sides of fillets, using all the spice mix.
3. Bake 10-13 minutes or until fish flakes easily with a fork. Serve.

Nutrition: Calories 366 Total Carbs 0g Protein 35g Fat 24g Sugar 0g Fiber 0g

201. Cajun Flounder & Tomatoes

Preparation time: 10 minutes
Cooking time: 15 minutes
Servings: 4
Ingredients:

- 4 flounder fillets
- 2 ½ cups tomatoes, diced
- ¾ cup onion, diced
- ¾ cup green bell pepper, diced
- What you'll need from store cupboard:
- 2 cloves garlic, diced fine
- 1 tbsp. Cajun seasoning
- 1 tsp olive oil

Directions:

1. Heat oil in a large skillet over med-high heat. Add onion and garlic and cook 2 minutes, or until soft. Add tomatoes, peppers and spices, and cook 2-3 minutes until tomatoes soften.
2. Lay fish over top. Cover, reduce heat to medium and cook, 5-8 minutes, or until fish flakes easily with a fork. Transfer fish to serving plates and top with sauce.

Nutrition: Calories 194 Total Carbs 8g Net Carbs 6g Protein 32g Fat 3g Sugar 5g Fiber 2g

202. Cajun Shrimp & Roasted Vegetables

Preparation time: 5 minutes
Cooking time: 15 minutes
Servings: 4
Ingredients:

- 1 lb. large shrimp, peeled and deveined
- 2 zucchinis, sliced
- 2 yellow squash, sliced
- ½ bunch asparagus, cut into thirds
- 2 red bell pepper, cut into chunks
- What you'll need from store cupboard:
- 2 tbsp. olive oil
- 2 tbsp. Cajun Seasoning
- Salt & pepper, to taste

Directions:

1. Heat oven to 400 degrees.
2. Combine shrimp and vegetables in a large bowl. Add oil and seasoning and toss to coat.
3. Spread evenly in a large baking sheet and bake 15-20 minutes, or until vegetables are tender. Serve.

Nutrition: Calories 251 Total Carbs 13g Net Carbs 9g Protein 30g Fat 9g Sugar 6g Fiber 4g

203. Cilantro Lime Grilled Shrimp

Preparation time: 5 minutes,
Cooking time: 5 minutes,
Servings: 6
Ingredients:

- 1 ½ lbs. large shrimp raw, peeled, deveined with tails on
- Juice and zest of 1 lime
- 2 tbsp. fresh cilantro chopped
- What you'll need from store cupboard:
- ¼ cup olive oil
- 2 cloves garlic, diced fine
- 1 tsp smoked paprika
- ¼ tsp cumin
- 1/2 teaspoon salt
- ¼ tsp cayenne pepper

Directions:

1. Place the shrimp in a large Ziploc bag.
2. Mix remaining Ingredients in a small bowl and pour over shrimp. Let marinate 20-30 minutes.
3. Heat up the grill. Skewer the shrimp and cook 2-3 minutes, per side, just until they turn pick. Be careful not to overcook them. Serve garnished with cilantro.

Nutrition: Calories 317 Total Carbs 4g Protein 39g Fat 15g Sugar 0g Fiber 0g

204. Crab Frittata

Preparation time: 10 minutes
Cooking time: 50 minutes
Servings: 4
Ingredients:

- 4 eggs
- 2 cups lump crabmeat
- 1 cup half-n-half
- 1 cup green onions, diced
- What you'll need from store cupboard:
- 1 cup reduced fat parmesan cheese, grated
- 1 tsp salt
- 1 tsp pepper
- 1 tsp smoked paprika
- 1 tsp Italian seasoning
- Nonstick cooking spray

Directions:

1. Heat oven to 350 degrees. Spray an 8-inch springform pan, or pie plate with cooking spray.
2. In a large bowl, whisk together the eggs and half-n-half. Add seasonings and parmesan cheese, stir to mix.
3. Stir in the onions and crab meat. Pour into prepared pan and bake 35-40 minutes, or eggs are set and top is lightly browned.
4. Let cool 10 minutes, then slice and serve warm or at room temperature.

Nutrition: Calories 276 Total Carbs 5g Net Carbs 4g Protein 25g Fat 17g Sugar 1g Fiber 1g

205. Crunchy Lemon Shrimp

Preparation time: 5 minutes
Cooking time: 10 minutes,
Servings: 4
Ingredients:

- 1 lb. raw shrimp, peeled and deveined
- 2 tbsp. Italian parsley, roughly chopped
- 2 tbsp. lemon juice, divided
- What you'll need from store cupboard:
- ⅔ cup panko bread crumbs
- 2½ tbsp. olive oil, divided
- Salt and pepper, to taste

Directions:

1. Heat oven to 400 degrees.
2. Place the shrimp evenly in a baking dish and sprinkle with salt and pepper. Drizzle on 1 tablespoon lemon juice and 1 tablespoon of olive oil. Set aside.
3. In a medium bowl, combine parsley, remaining lemon juice, bread crumbs, remaining olive oil, and ¼ tsp each of salt and pepper. Layer the panko mixture evenly on top of the shrimp.
4. Bake 8-10 minutes or until shrimp are cooked through and the panko is golden brown.

Nutrition: Calories 283 Total Carbs 15g Net Carbs 14g Protein 28g Fat 12g Sugar 1g Fiber 1g

206. Grilled Tuna Steaks

Preparation time: 5 minutes
Cooking time: 10 minutes,
Servings: 6
Ingredients:

- 6 6 oz. tuna steaks
- 3 tbsp. fresh basil, diced
- What you'll need from store cupboard:
- 4 ½ tsp olive oil

- ¾ tsp salt
- ¼ tsp pepper
- Nonstick cooking spray

Directions:
1. Heat grill to medium heat. Spray rack with cooking spray.
2. Drizzle both sides of the tuna with oil. Sprinkle with basil, salt and pepper.
3. Place on grill and cook 5 minutes per side, tuna should be slightly pink in the center. Serve.

Nutrition: Calories 343 Total Carbs 0g Protein 51g Fat 14g Sugar 0g Fiber 0g

207. Red Clam Sauce & Pasta

Preparation time: 10 minutes,
Cooking time: 3 hours,
Servings: 4
Ingredients:
- 1 onion, diced
- ¼ cup fresh parsley, diced
- What you'll need from store cupboard:
- 2 6 ½ oz. cans clams, chopped, undrained
- 14 ½ oz. tomatoes, diced, undrained
- 6 oz. tomato paste
- 2 cloves garlic, diced
- 1 bay leaf
- 1 tbsp. sunflower oil
- 1 tsp Splenda
- 1 tsp basil
- ½ tsp thyme
- ½ Homemade Pasta, cook & drain (chapter 15)

Directions:
1. Heat oil in a small skillet over med-high heat. Add onion and cook until tender, Add garlic and cook 1 minute more. Transfer to crock pot.
2. Add remaining Ingredients, except pasta, cover and cook on low 3-4 hours.
3. Discard bay leaf and serve over cooked pasta.

Nutrition: Calories 223 Total Carbs 32g Net Carbs 27g Protein 12g Fat 6g Sugar 15g Fiber 5g

208. Salmon Milano

Preparation time: 10 minutes,
Cooking time: 20 minutes,
Servings: 6
Ingredients:
- 2 ½ lb. salmon filet
- 2 tomatoes, sliced
- ½ cup margarine
- What you'll need from store cupboard:
- ½ cup basil pesto

Directions:
1. Heat the oven to 400 degrees. Line a 9x15-inch baking sheet with foil, making sure it covers the sides. Place another large piece of foil onto the baking sheet and place the salmon filet on top of it.
2. Place the pesto and margarine in blender or food processor and pulse until smooth. Spread evenly over salmon. Place tomato slices on top.

3. Wrap the foil around the salmon, tenting around the top to prevent foil from touching the salmon as much as possible. Bake 15-25 minutes, or salmon flakes easily with a fork. Serve.

Nutrition: Calories 444 Total Carbs 2g Protein 55g Fat 24g Sugar 1g Fiber 0g

209. Shrimp & Artichoke Skillet

Preparation time: 5 minutes
Cooking time: 10 minutes
Servings: 4
Ingredients:
- 1 ½ cups shrimp, peel & devein
- 2 shallots, diced
- 1 tbsp. margarine
- What you'll need from store cupboard
- 2 12 oz. jars artichoke hearts, drain & rinse
- 2 cups white wine
- 2 cloves garlic, diced fine

Directions:
1. Melt margarine in a large skillet over med-high heat. Add shallot and garlic and cook until they start to brown, stirring frequently.
2. Add artichokes and cook 5 minutes. Reduce heat and add wine. Cook 3 minutes, stirring occasionally.
3. Add the shrimp and cook just until they turn pink. Serve.

Nutrition: Calories 487 Total Carbs 26g Net Carbs 17g Protein 64g Fat 5g Sugar 3g Fiber 9g

210. Tuna Carbonara

Preparation time: 5 minutes
Cooking time: 25 minutes
Servings: 4
Ingredients:
- ½ lb. tuna fillet, cut in pieces
- 2 eggs
- 4 tbsp. fresh parsley, diced
- What you'll need from store cupboard:
- ½ Homemade Pasta, cook & drain, (chapter 15)
- ½ cup reduced fat parmesan cheese
- 2 cloves garlic, peeled
- 2 tbsp. extra virgin olive oil
- Salt & pepper, to taste

Directions:
1. In a small bowl, beat the eggs, parmesan and a dash of pepper.
2. Heat the oil in a large skillet over med-high heat. Add garlic and cook until browned. Add the tuna and cook 2-3 minutes, or until tuna is almost cooked through. Discard the garlic.
3. Add the pasta and reduce heat. Stir in egg mixture and cook, stirring constantly, 2 minutes. If the sauce is too thick, thin with water, a little bit at a time, until it has a creamy texture.
4. Salt and pepper to taste and serve garnished with parsley.

Nutrition: Calories 409 Total Carbs 7g Net Carbs 6g Protein 25g Fat 30g Sugar 3g Fiber 1g

211. Mediterranean Fish Fillets

Preparation Time: 10 minutes
Cooking Time: 3 minutes
Servings: 4
Ingredients:

- 4 cod fillets
- 1 lb grape tomatoes, halved
- 1 cup olives, pitted and sliced
- 2 tbsp capers
- 1 tsp dried thyme
- 2 tbsp olive oil
- 1 tsp garlic, minced
- Pepper
- Salt

Directions:

1. Pour 1 cup water into the instant pot then place steamer rack in the pot.
2. Spray heat-safe baking dish with cooking spray.
3. Add half grape tomatoes into the dish and season with pepper and salt.
4. Arrange fish fillets on top of cherry tomatoes. Drizzle with oil and season with garlic, thyme, capers, pepper, and salt.
5. Spread olives and remaining grape tomatoes on top of fish fillets.
6. Place dish on top of steamer rack in the pot.
7. Seal pot with a lid and select manual and cook on high for 3 minutes.
8. Once done, release pressure using quick release. Remove lid.
9. Serve and enjoy.

Nutrition: Calories 212 Fat 11.9 g Carbohydrates 7.1 g Sugar 3 g Protein 21.4 g Cholesterol 55 mg

212. Flavors Cioppino

Preparation Time: 10 minutes
Cooking Time: 5 minutes
Servings: 6
Ingredients:

- 1 lb codfish, cut into chunks
- 1 1/2 lbs shrimp
- 28 oz can tomatoes, diced
- 1 cup dry white wine
- 1 bay leaf
- 1 tsp cayenne
- 1 tsp oregano
- 1 shallot, chopped
- 1 tsp garlic, minced
- 1 tbsp olive oil
- 1/2 tsp salt

Directions:

1. Add oil into the inner pot of instant pot and set the pot on sauté mode.
2. Add shallot and garlic and sauté for 2 minutes.
3. Add wine, bay leaf, cayenne, oregano, and salt and cook for 3 minutes.
4. Add remaining ingredients and stir well.

5. Seal pot with a lid and select manual and cook on low for 0 minutes.
6. Once done, release pressure using quick release. Remove lid.
7. Serve and enjoy.

Nutrition: Calories 281 Fat 5 g Carbohydrates 10.5 g Sugar 4.9 g Protein 40.7 g Cholesterol 266 mg

213. Delicious Shrimp Alfredo

Preparation Time: 10 minutes
Cooking Time: 3 minutes
Servings: 4
Ingredients:

- 12 shrimp, remove shells
- 1 tbsp garlic, minced
- 1/4 cup parmesan cheese
- 2 cups whole wheat rotini noodles
- 1 cup fish broth
- 15 oz alfredo sauce
- 1 onion, chopped
- Salt

Directions:

1. Add all ingredients except parmesan cheese into the instant pot and stir well.
2. Seal pot with lid and cook on high for 3 minutes.
3. Once done, release pressure using quick release. Remove lid.
4. Stir in cheese and serve.

Nutrition: Calories 669 Fat 23.1 g Carbohydrates 76 g Sugar 2.4 g Protein 37.8 g Cholesterol 190 mg

214. Tomato Olive Fish Fillets

Preparation Time: 10 minutes
Cooking Time: 8 minutes
Servings: 4
Ingredients:

- 2 lbs halibut fish fillets
- 2 oregano sprigs
- 2 rosemary sprigs
- 2 tbsp fresh lime juice
- 1 cup olives, pitted
- 28 oz can tomatoes, diced
- 1 tbsp garlic, minced
- 1 onion, chopped
- 2 tbsp olive oil

Directions:

1. Add oil into the inner pot of instant pot and set the pot on sauté mode.
2. Add onion and sauté for 3 minutes.
3. Add garlic and sauté for a minute.
4. Add lime juice, olives, herb sprigs, and tomatoes and stir well.
5. Seal pot with lid and cook on high for 3 minutes.
6. Once done, release pressure using quick release. Remove lid.
7. Add fish fillets and seal pot again with lid and cook on high for 2 minutes.
8. Once done, release pressure using quick release. Remove lid.
9. Serve and enjoy.

Nutrition: Calories 333 Fat 19.1 g Carbohydrates 31.8 g Sugar 8.4 g Protein 13.4 g Cholesterol 5 mg

215. Easy Salmon Stew

Preparation Time: 10 minutes
Cooking Time: 8 minutes
Servings: 6
Ingredients:

- 2 lbs salmon fillet, cubed
- 1 onion, chopped
- 2 cups fish broth
- 1 tbsp olive oil
- Pepper
- salt

Directions:

1. Add oil into the inner pot of instant pot and set the pot on sauté mode.
2. Add onion and sauté for 2 minutes.
3. Add remaining ingredients and stir well.
4. Seal pot with lid and cook on high for 6 minutes.
5. Once done, release pressure using quick release. Remove lid.
6. Stir and serve.

Nutrition: Calories 243 Fat 12.6 g Carbohydrates 0.8 g Sugar 0.3 g Protein 31 g Cholesterol 78 mg

216. Italian Tuna Pasta

Preparation Time: 10 minutes
Cooking Time: 5 minutes
Servings: 6
Ingredients:

- 15 oz whole wheat pasta
- 2 tbsp capers
- 3 oz tuna
- 2 cups can tomatoes, crushed
- 2 anchovies
- 1 tsp garlic, minced
- 1 tbsp olive oil
- Salt

Directions:

1. Add oil into the inner pot of instant pot and set the pot on sauté mode.
2. Add anchovies and garlic and sauté for 1 minute.
3. Add remaining ingredients and stir well. Pour enough water into the pot to cover the pasta.
4. Seal pot with a lid and select manual and cook on low for 4 minutes.
5. Once done, release pressure using quick release. Remove lid.
6. Stir and serve.

Nutrition: Calories 339 Fat 6 g Carbohydrates 56.5 g Sugar 5.2 g Protein 15.2 g Cholesterol 10 mg

217. Garlicky Clams

Preparation Time: 10 minutes
Cooking Time: 5 minutes
Servings: 4
Ingredients:

- 3 lbs clams, clean
- 4 garlic cloves

- 1/4 cup olive oil
- 1/2 cup fresh lemon juice
- 1 cup white wine
- Pepper
- Salt

Directions:

1. Add oil into the inner pot of instant pot and set the pot on sauté mode.
2. Add garlic and sauté for 1 minute.
3. Add wine and cook for 2 minutes.
4. Add remaining ingredients and stir well.
5. Seal pot with lid and cook on high for 2 minutes.
6. Once done, allow to release pressure naturally. Remove lid.
7. Serve and enjoy.

Nutrition: Calories 332 Fat 13.5 g Carbohydrates 40.5 g Sugar 12.4 g Protein 2.5 g Cholesterol 0 mg

218. Delicious Fish Tacos

Preparation Time: 10 minutes
Cooking Time: 8 minutes
Servings: 8
Ingredients:

- 4 tilapia fillets
- 1/4 cup fresh cilantro, chopped
- 1/4 cup fresh lime juice
- 2 tbsp paprika
- 1 tbsp olive oil
- Pepper
- Salt

Directions:

1. Pour 2 cups of water into the instant pot then place steamer rack in the pot.
2. Place fish fillets on parchment paper.
3. Season fish fillets with paprika, pepper, and salt and drizzle with oil and lime juice.
4. Fold parchment paper around the fish fillets and place them on a steamer rack in the pot.
5. Seal pot with lid and cook on high for 8 minutes.
6. Once done, release pressure using quick release. Remove lid.
7. Remove fish packet from pot and open it.
8. Shred the fish with a fork and serve.

Nutrition: Calories 67 Fat 2.5 g Carbohydrates 1.1 g Sugar 0.2 g Protein 10.8 g Cholesterol 28 mg

219. Pesto Fish Fillet

Preparation Time: 10 minutes
Cooking Time: 8 minutes
Servings: 4
Ingredients:

- 4 halibut fillets
- 1/2 cup water
- 1 tbsp lemon zest, grated
- 1 tbsp capers
- 1/2 cup basil, chopped
- 1 tbsp garlic, chopped
- 1 avocado, peeled and chopped
- Pepper

- Salt

Directions:
1. Add lemon zest, capers, basil, garlic, avocado, pepper, and salt into the blender blend until smooth.
2. Place fish fillets on aluminum foil and spread a blended mixture on fish fillets.
3. Fold foil around the fish fillets.
4. Pour water into the instant pot and place trivet in the pot.
5. Place foil fish packet on the trivet.
6. Seal pot with lid and cook on high for 8 minutes.
7. Once done, allow to release pressure naturally. Remove lid.
8. Serve and enjoy.

Nutrition: Calories 426 Fat 16.6 g Carbohydrates 5.5 g Sugar 0.4 g Protein 61.8 g Cholesterol 93 mg

220. **Salsa Fish Fillets**

Preparation Time: 10 minutes
Cooking Time: 2 minutes
Servings: 4
Ingredients:
- 1 lb tilapia fillets
- 1/2 cup salsa
- 1 cup of water
- Pepper
- Salt

Directions:
1. Place fish fillets on aluminum foil and top with salsa and season with pepper and salt.
2. Fold foil around the fish fillets.
3. Pour water into the instant pot and place trivet in the pot.
4. Place foil fish packet on the trivet.
5. Seal pot with lid and cook on high for 2 minutes.
6. Once done, release pressure using quick release. Remove lid.
7. Serve and enjoy.

Nutrition: Calories 342 Fat 10.5 g Carbohydrates 41.5 g Sugar 1.9 g Protein 18.9 g Cholesterol 31 mg

221. **Coconut Clam Chowder**

Preparation Time: 10 minutes
Cooking Time: 7 minutes
Servings: 6
Ingredients:
- 6 oz clams, chopped
- 1 cup heavy cream
- 1/4 onion, sliced
- 1 cup celery, chopped
- 1 lb cauliflower, chopped
- 1 cup fish broth
- 1 bay leaf
- 2 cups of coconut milk
- Salt

Directions:
1. Add all ingredients except clams and heavy cream and stir well.
2. Seal pot with lid and cook on high for 5 minutes.

3. Once done, release pressure using quick release. Remove lid.
4. Add heavy cream and clams and stir well and cook on sauté mode for 2 minutes.
5. Stir well and serve.

Nutrition: Calories 301 Fat 27.2 g Carbohydrates 13.6 g Sugar 6 g Protein 4.9 g Cholesterol 33 mg

222. **Almond Crusted Baked Chili Mahi**

Preparation Time: 20 minutes
Cooking Time: 15 minutes
Servings: 8
Ingredients:
- 4 Mahi fillets
- 1 lime
- 2 teaspoons olive oil
- Salt and pepper to taste
- ½ cup almonds
- ¼ teaspoon paprika
- ¼ teaspoon onion powder
- ¾ teaspoon chili powder
- ½ cup red bell pepper, chopped
- ¼ cup onion, chopped
- ¼ cup fresh cilantro, chopped

Directions:
1. Preheat your oven to 325 degrees F.
2. Line your baking pan with parchment paper.
3. Squeeze juice from the lime.
4. Grate zest from the peel.
5. Put juice and zest in a bowl.
6. Add the oil, salt and pepper.
7. In another bowl, add the almonds, paprika, onion powder and chili powder.
8. Put the almond mixture in a food processor.
9. Pulse until powdery.
10. Dip each fillet in the oil mixture.
11. Dredge with the almond and chili mixture.
12. Arrange on a single layer in the oven.
13. Bake for 12 to 15 minutes or until fully cooked.
14. Serve with red bell pepper, onion and cilantro.

Nutrition: Calories 105 Fat 27.2 g Carbohydrates 13.6 g Protein 4.3 g Cholesterol 31 mg

223. **Swordfish with Tomato Salsa**

Preparation Time: 20 minutes
Cooking Time: 12 minutes
Servings: 4
Ingredients:
- 1 cup tomato, chopped
- ¼ cup tomatillo, chopped
- 2 tablespoons fresh cilantro, chopped
- ¼ cup avocado, chopped
- 1 clove garlic, minced
- 1 jalapeño pepper, chopped
- 1 tablespoon lime juice
- Salt and pepper to taste
- 4 swordfish steaks

- 1 clove garlic, sliced in half
- 2 tablespoons lemon juice
- ½ teaspoon ground cumin

Directions:

1. Preheat your grill.
2. In a bowl, mix the tomato, tomatillo, cilantro, avocado, garlic, jalapeño, lime juice, salt and pepper.
3. Cover the bowl with foil and put in the refrigerator.
4. Rub each swordfish steak with sliced garlic.
5. Drizzle lemon juice on both sides.
6. Season with salt, pepper and cumin.
7. Grill for 12 minutes or until the fish is fully cooked.
8. Serve with salsa.

Nutrition: Calories 125 g Fat 27.2 g Carbohydrates 13.6 g Protein 7 g Cholesterol 31 mg

224. Salmon & Asparagus

Preparation Time: 10 minutes
Cooking Time: 10 minutes
Servings: 2
Ingredients:

- 2 salmon fillets
- 8 spears asparagus, trimmed
- 2 tablespoons balsamic vinegar
- 1 teaspoon olive oil
- 1 teaspoon dried dill
- Salt and pepper to taste

Directions:

1. Preheat your oven to 325 degrees F.
2. Dry salmon with paper towels.
3. Arrange the asparagus around the salmon fillets on a baking pan.
4. In a bowl, mix the rest of the ingredients.
5. Pour mixture over the salmon and vegetables.
6. Bake in the oven for 10 minutes or until the fish is fully cooked.

Nutrition: Calories 150 g Fat 22 g Carbohydrates 13.6 g Protein 7 g Cholesterol 20 mg

225. Halibut with Spicy Apricot Sauce

Preparation Time: 20 minutes
Cooking Time: 17 minutes
Servings: 4
Ingredients:

- 4 fresh apricots, pitted
- ⅓ cup apricot preserves
- ½ cup apricot nectar
- ½ teaspoon dried oregano
- 3 tablespoons scallion, sliced
- 1 teaspoon hot pepper sauce
- Salt to taste
- 4 halibut steaks
- 1 tablespoon olive oil

Directions:

1. Put the apricots, preserves, nectar, oregano, scallion, hot pepper sauce and salt in a saucepan.

2. Bring to a boil and then simmer for 8 minutes.
3. Set aside.
4. Brush the halibut steaks with olive oil.
5. Grill for 7 to 9 minutes or until fish is flaky.
6. Brush one tablespoon of the sauce on both sides of the fish.
7. Serve with the reserved sauce.
8. Bake in the oven for 10 minutes or until the fish is fully cooked.

Nutrition: Calories 150 g Fat 22 g Carbohydrates 13.6 g Protein 7 g Cholesterol 20 mg

226. Popcorn Shrimp

Preparation Time: 10 minutes
Cooking Time: 8 minutes
Servings: 4
Ingredients:

- Cooking spray
- ½ cup all-purpose flour
- 2 eggs, beaten
- 2 tablespoons water
- 1 ½ cups panko breadcrumbs
- 1 tablespoon garlic powder
- 1 tablespoon ground cumin
- 1 lb. shrimp, peeled and deveined
- ½ cup ketchup
- 2 tablespoons fresh cilantro, chopped
- 2 tablespoons lime juice
- Salt to taste

Directions:

1. Coat the air fryer basket with cooking spray
2. Put the flour in a dish.
3. In the second dish, beat the eggs and water.
4. In the third dish, mix the breadcrumbs, garlic powder and cumin.
5. Dip each shrimp in each of the three dishes, first in the dish with flour, then the egg and then breadcrumb mixture.
6. Place the shrimp in the air fryer basket.
7. Cook at 360 degrees F for 8 minutes, flipping once halfway through.
8. Combine the rest of the ingredients as dipping sauce for the shrimp.

Nutrition: Calories 200 g Fat 25 g Carbohydrates 13.8 g Protein 10 g Cholesterol 21 mg

227. Shrimp Lemon Kebab

Preparation Time: 10 minutes
Cooking Time: 4 minutes
Servings: 5
Ingredients:

- 1 ½ lb. shrimp, peeled and deveined but with tails intact
- ⅓ cup olive oil
- ¼ cup lemon juice
- 2 teaspoons lemon zest
- 1 tablespoon fresh parsley, chopped
- 8 cherry tomatoes, quartered

- 2 scallions, sliced

Directions:

1. Mix the olive oil, lemon juice, lemon zest and parsley in a bowl.
2. Marinate the shrimp in this mixture for 15 minutes.
3. Thread each shrimp into the skewers.
4. Grill for 4 to 5 minutes, turning once halfway through.
5. Serve with tomatoes and scallions.

Nutrition: Calories 180 g Fat 20 g Carbohydrates 15 g Protein 11 g Cholesterol 26 mg

228. Grilled Herbed Salmon with Raspberry Sauce & Cucumber Dill Dip

Preparation Time: 20 minutes
Cooking Time: 30 minutes
Servings: 4
Ingredients:

- 3 salmon fillets
- 1 tablespoon olive oil
- Salt and pepper to taste
- 1 teaspoon fresh sage, chopped
- 1 tablespoon fresh parsley, chopped
- 2 tablespoons apple juice
- 1 cup raspberries
- 1 teaspoon Worcestershire sauce
- 1 cup cucumber, chopped
- 2 tablespoons light mayonnaise
- ½ teaspoon dried dill

Directions:

1. Coat the salmon fillets with oil.
2. Season with salt, pepper, sage and parsley.
3. Cover the salmon with foil.
4. Grill for 20 minutes or until fish is flaky.
5. While waiting, mix the apple juice, raspberries and Worcestershire sauce.
6. Pour the mixture into a saucepan over medium heat.
7. Bring to a boil and then simmer for 8 minutes.
8. In another bowl, mix the rest of the ingredients.
9. Serve salmon with raspberry sauce and cucumber dip.

Nutrition: Calories 301 Fat 27.2 g Carbohydrates 13.6 g Protein 4.9 g Cholesterol 33 mg

229. Tarragon Scallops

Preparation Time: 20 minutes
Cooking Time: 15 minutes
Servings: 4
Ingredients:

- 1 cup water
- 1 lb. asparagus spears, trimmed
- 2 lemons
- 1 ¼ lb. scallops
- Salt and pepper to taste

- 1 tablespoon olive oil
- 1 tablespoon fresh tarragon, chopped

Directions:

1. Pour water into a pot.
2. Bring to a boil.
3. Add asparagus spears.
4. Cover and cook for 5 minutes.
5. Drain and transfer to a plate.
6. Slice one lemon into wedges.
7. Squeeze juice and shred zest from the remaining lemon.
8. Season the scallops with salt and pepper.
9. Put a pan over medium heat.
10. Add oil to the pan.
11. Cook the scallops until golden brown.
12. Transfer to the same plate, putting scallops beside the asparagus.
13. Add lemon zest, juice and tarragon to the pan.
14. Cook for 1 minute.
15. Drizzle tarragon sauce over the scallops and asparagus.

Nutrition: Calories 250 g Fat 10 g Carbohydrates 30 g Protein 15 g Cholesterol 24 mg

230. Garlic Shrimp & Spinach

Preparation Time: 20 minutes
Cooking Time: 30 minutes
Servings: 4
Ingredients:

- 3 tablespoons olive oil, divided
- 6 clove garlic, sliced and divided
- 1 lb. spinach
- Salt to taste
- 1 tablespoons lemon juice
- 1 lb. shrimp, peeled and deveined
- ¼ teaspoon red pepper, crushed
- 1 tablespoon parsley, chopped
- 1 teaspoon lemon zest

Directions:

1. Pour 1 tablespoon olive oil in a pot over medium heat.
2. Cook the garlic for 1 minute.
3. Add the spinach and season with salt.
4. Cook for 3 minutes.
5. Stir in lemon juice.
6. Transfer to a bowl.
7. Pour the remaining oil.
8. Add the shrimp.
9. Season with salt and add red pepper.
10. Cook for 5 minutes.
11. Sprinkle parsley and lemon zest over the shrimp before serving.

Nutrition: Calories 280 g Fat 10 g Carbohydrates 35 g Protein 15 g Cholesterol 24 mg

POULTRY RECIPES

231. Slow-Cooker Chicken Fajita Burritos

Preparation time: 10 minutes
Cooking Time: 6 hrs
Servings: 8
Ingredients:

- 1 teaspoon cumin
- 1 cup cheddar cheese + 2 tablespoons reduced-fat, shredded
- 1 lb. chicken strips, skinless and boneless
- 8 large low-carb tortillas
- 1 green pepper, sliced
- 1 can (15 oz) black beans, rinsed and drained
- 1 red pepper, sliced
- 1/3 cup water
- 1 medium onion, sliced
- ½ cup salsa
- 1 tablespoon chili powder
- 1 teaspoon garlic powder

Directions:

1. Place strips of chicken breast in a slow-cooker.
2. Top chicken with all ingredients mentioned above except for cheese and tortillas. Cover the cooker and cook for approximately 6 hours, until done.
3. Shred chicken with a fork.
4. Serve half cup of chicken on each tortilla along with the bean mixture.
5. Finish with 2 tablespoons of shredded cheese, then fold tortilla into a burrito.

Nutrition: 250 calories; 7 g fat; 31 g total carbs; 28 g protein

232. Crock Pot Chicken Cacciatore

Preparation time: 10 minutes
Cooking time: 4 hours
Servings: 6
Ingredients:

- 1 can (14.5 oz) tomatoes, diced
- 6 medium chicken thighs, skins removed
- 1 onion, sliced
- 1 tablespoon Italian seasoning
- 1 green bell pepper, seeded and sliced
- 3 clove garlic, minced
- 2 can (6-oz, no salt added) tomato paste

Directions:

1. To a Crock-Pot slow cooker, add all ingredients and cook for 4 hours on High.
2. Once done, serve chicken cacciatore with whole wheat rotini pasta, if desired.

Nutrition: 170 calories; 5 g fat; 18 g total carbs; 16 g protein

233. Crock-Pot Slow Cooker Chicken & Sweet Potatoes

Preparation time: 10 minutes
Cooking time: 5-7 hours
Servings: 4

Ingredients:

- 1 1/2 cup low-sodium and low-fat chicken broth
- 1 bay leave
- 4 (4 oz) chicken thighs, skinless and boneless
- 2 tablespoons Dijon mustard
- 1 onion, chopped
- ¼ teaspoon dried thyme
- 2 large sweet potatoes, peeled and sliced into large rounds
- 3 tablespoons Splenda Brown Sugar blend

Directions:

1. Place 4 (4 oz) chicken thighs into the Crock-Pot slow cooker.
2. Top chicken thighs with sliced potatoes and chopped onions.
3. Now add all leftover ingredients to the Crock-Pot slow cooker. Cook for about 5-7 hours on low until chicken is completely cooked through.
4. Once done, remove bay leaf from the Crock-Pot slow cooker.
5. Serve right away.

Nutrition: 75 calories; 7 g fat; 32 g total carbs; 21 g protein

234. Crock-Pot Slow Cooker Tex-Mex Chicken

Preparation time: 10 minutes
Cooking time: 4 hours 40 minutes
Servings: 6
Ingredients:

- 4 tablespoons cup water
- 1 teaspoon ground cumin
- 1 lb boneless chicken thighs, visible fat removed, rinsed, and patted dry
- 1 (10 oz) can diced tomatoes and green chilies
- 1 (16 oz) package frozen onion and pepper strips, thawed

Directions:

1. Spray a skillet with cooking spray and turn heat flame on.
2. Place chicken thighs into the skillet and cook each side until browned over medium heat. Once browned, take out from the skillet.
3. To the same skillet, add peppers and onions and cook until tender.
4. Transfer cooked peppers and onions into 4- to 5-quart Crock-Pot slow cooker followed by chicken thighs on top.
5. Place tomatoes along with 4 tablespoons of water over chicken. Cook for about 4 hours on Low.
6. Add 1 teaspoon ground cumin and cook further for half an hour.
7. Once done, take it out and serve right away!

Nutrition: 121 calories; 3.2 g fat; 6.4 g total carbs; 16 g protein

235. Crock-Pot Slow Cooker Ranch Chicken

Preparation time: 10 minutes
Cooking time: 4 hours
Servings: 4
Ingredients:

- 1 cup chive and onion cream cheese spread
- ½ teaspoon freshly ground black pepper
- 4 boneless chicken breasts
- 1 1-oz package ranch dressing and seasoning mix
- ½ cup low sodium chicken stock

Directions:

1. Spray the Crock-Pot slow cooker with cooking spray and preheat it.
2. Dry chicken with paper towel and transfer it to the Crock-Pot slow cooker.
3. Cook each side, until chicken is browned, for about 4-5 minutes.
4. Add ½ cup low sodium chicken stock, 1 1-oz. package ranch dressing and seasoning mix, 1 cup chive and onion cream cheese spread and ½ teaspoon freshly ground black pepper. Cover the Crock-Pot slow cooker and cook for about 4 hours on Low or until the internal temperature reaches 165 F. Once cooked, take it out from the Crock-Pot slow cooker.
5. Whisk the sauce present in the Crock-Pot slow cooker until smooth. If you need thick sauce, then cook for about 5-10 minutes, with frequent stirring.
6. Garnish chicken with sliced onions and bacon and serve.

Nutrition: 362 calories; 18.5 g fat; 9.7 g total carbs; 37.3 g protein

236. Crock-Pot Buffalo Chicken Dip

Preparation time: 10 minutes
Cooking time: 3 hours
Servings: 10
Ingredients:

- 2 cups cooked chicken, chopped into small pieces
- 1 cup ranch dressing
- 16 oz cream cheese, cubed and softened
- 5 ounces' hot sauce

Directions:

1. add 5 oz hot sauce, 16 ounces cubed cream cheese, and 1 cup ranch dressing to a 3-quart Crock-Pot slow cooker. Cover it and cook for about 2 hours on Low, with occasional stirring.
2. Once cheese is melted, add 2 cups of cooked chicken. Cover the Crock-Pot slow cooker again and cook again for 1 hour on Low.
3. Serve buffalo chicken along with veggies or any of your favorite chips.

Nutrition: 344 calories; 29 g fat; 5 g total carbs; 15 g protein

237. Crock-Pot Slow Cooker Mulligatawny Soup

Preparation time: 10 minutes
Cooking time: 6 hours
Servings: 8
Ingredients:

- 2 whole cloves
- 1/4 cup green pepper, chopped
- 1 carton (32 oz.) low-sodium chicken broth
- 1/4 teaspoon pepper
- 1 can (14 1/2 oz.) diced tomatoes
- 1/2 teaspoon sugar
- 2 cups cubed cooked chicken
- 1 teaspoon curry powder
- 1 large tart green apple, peeled and chopped
- 1 teaspoon salt
- 1/4 cup onion, finely chopped
- 2 teaspoon lemon juice
- 1/4 cup carrot, chopped
- 1 tablespoon fresh parsley, minced

Directions:

1. Add all ingredients in a 3- or 4-qt. Crock-Pot slow cooker and combine well. Cover the cooker and cook for about 6-8 hours on Low.
2. Once done, remove cloves and serve.

Nutrition: 107 calories; 2 g fat; 10 g total carbs; 12 g protein

238. Greek Chicken

Preparation time: 10 minutes
Cooking time: 9-10 hours
Servings: 4-6
Ingredients:

- 1 whole bulb garlic, minced
- 1 tablespoon olive oil
- 4 potatoes, unpeeled and quartered
- 1/2 teaspoon pepper
- 2 pounds chicken pieces, trimmed of skin and fat
- 3/4 teaspoon salt
- 2 large onions, quartered
- 3 teaspoons dried oregano

Directions:

1. Add potatoes into the slow cooker, spread on the bottom.
2. The add 2 pounds' chicken pieces along with minced garlic and quartered onions.
3. Sprinkle with 3 teaspoons dried oregano, 3/4 teaspoon salt, and 1/2 teaspoon pepper.
4. Drizzle with 1 tablespoon olive oil.
5. Cook for about 9-10 hours on low and 5-6 hours on high.

Nutrition: 278 calories; 6 g fat; 29 g total carbs; 27 g protein

239. Polynesian Chicken

Preparation time: 10 minutes
Cooking time: 4 hours
Servings: 6 cups
Ingredients:

- 3 garlic cloves, minced
- 2 bell peppers, cut into 1/2-inch strips
- 1 (20-ounce) can pineapple chunks in juice, drained, with juice reserved
- 1 1/2-pound boneless chicken breasts, cut into 2-inch cubes

- 1/3 cup honey
- 2 tablespoons tapioca flour
- 3 tablespoons low-sodium soy sauce
- 1 teaspoon ground ginger

Directions:

1. Add reserved pineapple juice, 3 tablespoons of soy sauce, 1/3 cup honey, 1 teaspoon ground ginger and 3 minced cloves of garlic into a bowl; whisk well. Then add 2 tablespoons tapioca flour and whisk again until combined.
2. Add chicken along with chunks of pineapple into a slow cooker.
3. Pour mixture of pineapple juice over chicken and cover the cooker.
4. Cook for about 4-5 hours on low, until chicken is completely cooked through.
5. Then add strips of bell pepper in the last hour of cooking. Serve and enjoy!

Nutrition: 273 calories; 26 g fat; 37 g total carbs; 26 g protein

240. Coconut Chicken

Preparation time: 10 minutes
Cooking time: 4 hours
Servings: 6
Ingredients:

- 2 garlic cloves, minced
- Fresh cilantro, minced
- 1/2 cup light coconut milk
- 6 tablespoons sweetened coconut, shredded and toasted
- 2 tablespoons brown sugar
- 6 (about 1-1/2 pounds) boneless skinless chicken thighs
- 2 tablespoons reduced-sodium soy sauce
- 1/8 teaspoon ground cloves

Directions:

1. Mix brown sugar, 1/2 cup light coconut milk, 2 tablespoons soy sauce, 1/8 teaspoon ground cloves and 2 minced cloves of garlic in a bowl.
2. Add 6 chicken boneless thighs into a Crockpot.
3. Now pour the mixture of coconut milk over chicken thighs. Cover the cooker and cook for about 4-5 hours on low.
4. Serve coconut chicken with cilantro and coconut; enjoy!

Nutrition: 201 calories; 10 g fat; 6 g total carbs; 21 g protein

241. Spicy Lime Chicken

Preparation time: 10 minutes
Cooking time: 3 hours
Servings: 6
Ingredients:

- 3 tablespoons lime juice
- Fresh cilantro leaves
- 1-1/2 pounds (about 4) boneless skinless chicken breast halves
- 1 teaspoon lime zest, grated
- 2 cups chicken broth

- 1 tablespoon chili powder

Directions:

1. Add chicken breast halves into a slow cooker.
2. Add 1 tablespoon chili powder, 3 tablespoons lime juice and 2 cups chicken broth in a small bowl; mix well and pour over chicken.
3. Cover the cooker and cook for about 3 hours on low. Once done, take chicken out from the cooker and let it cool.
4. Once cooled, shred chicken by using forks and transfer back to the Crockpot.
5. Stir in 1 teaspoon grated lime zest. Serve spicy lime chicken with cilantro and enjoy!

Nutrition: 132 calories; 3 g fat; 2 g total carbs; 23 g protein

242. Chuck and Veggies

Preparation time: 10 minutes
Cooking time: 9 hours
Servings: 2
Ingredients:

- ¼ cup dry red wine
- ¼ teaspoon salt
- 8 oz. boneless lean chuck roast
- ¼ teaspoon black pepper
- 8 oz. frozen pepper stir-fry
- 1 teaspoon Worcestershire sauce
- 8 oz. whole mushrooms
- 1 teaspoon instant coffee granules
- 1 1/4 cups fresh green beans, trimmed
- 1 dried bay leaf

Directions:

1. Mix all the ingredients except salt in a bowl; combine well and then transfer to a slow cooker.
2. Cover the cooker and cook for about 9 hours on low and 4 1/2 hours on high, until beef is completely cooked through and tender.
3. Stir in ¼ teaspoon salt gently. Take out the vegetables and beef and transfer to 2 shallow bowls.
4. Pour liquid into the skillet; boil it lightly and cook until liquid reduces to ¼ cup, for about 1 1/2 minutes.
5. Pour over veggies and beef. Discard bay leaf and serve.

Nutrition: 215 calories; 5 g fat; 17 g total carbs; 26 g protein

243. Mustard Chicken with Basil

Preparation Time: 20 minutes
Cooking Time: 30 minutes
Servings: 4
Ingredients:

- 1 tsp Chicken stock
- 2 Chicken breasts; skinless and boneless chicken breasts: halved
- 1 tbsp Chopped basil
- What you'll need from the store cupboard:
- Salt and black pepper
- 1 tbsp Olive oil
- ½ tsp Garlic powder
- ½ tsp Onion powder

- 1 tsp Dijon mustard

Directions:

1. Press 'Sauté' on the instant pot and add the oil. When it is hot, brown the chicken in it for 2-3 minutes.
2. Mix in the remaining ingredients and seal the lid to cook for 12 minutes at high pressure.
3. Natural release the pressure for 10 minutes, share into plates and serve.

Nutrition: Calories 34, fat 3.6, carbs 0.7, protein 0.3, fiber 0.1

244. **Basil Chili Chicken**

Preparation Time: 5 minutes
Cooking Time: 20 minutes
Servings: 4
Ingredients:

- half cup Chicken stock
- 1 lb. Chicken breast
- 2 tsp Sweet paprika
- 1 cup Coconut cream
- 2 tbsp Basil (sliced)
- What you'll need from the store cupboard:
- Salt and Black pepper to taste
- 1 tbsp Chili powder

Directions:

1. In your instant pot, mix the chicken with the other ingredients, then stir them a little, then cover them then heat for 20 minutes on high temperature.
2. Release the pressure gradually for 10 minutes then split them among plates before you eat them.

Nutrition: Calories: 364, Fat: 23.2, Fiber: 2.3g, Carbs: 5.1g, Protein: 35.4g

245. **Garlic Chives Chicken**

Preparation Time: 20 minutes
Cooking Time: 10 minutes
Servings: 4
Ingredients:

- 1 lb. (no skin and bones) Chicken breast
- 1 tbsp Chives
- 1 cup Chicken stock
- 1 cup Coconut cream
- 3 tbsp Garlic cloves (sliced)
- What you'll need from the store cupboard:
- 1 and a half tbsp Balsamic vinegar
- Salt and Black pepper to taste

Directions:

1. In the instant pot, mix the chicken with all the remaining ingredients, then cover them and cook for 20 minutes on high temperature.
2. Release the pressure gradually for 10 minutes then split them among your plates before eating.

Nutrition: Calories: 360, Fat: 22.1, Fiber: 1.4g, Carbs: 4.1g, Protein: 34.5g

246. **Turkey and Spring Onions Mix**

Preparation Time: 15 minutes
Cooking Time: 10 minutes
Servings: 4

Ingredients:

- Cilantro
- 4 pieces Spring onions (sliced)
- 1 piece (no skin and bones) Turkey breast
- 1 cup Tomato passata
- What you'll need from the store cupboard:
- 2 tbsp Avocado oil
- Salt and Black pepper to taste

Directions:

1. Put the instant pot on Sauté option, then put the oil and cook it. After that, put the meat then heat it for 5 minutes.
2. Put the other ingredients, then cover it and heat it for 20 minutes on high temperature.
3. Release the pressure gradually for 10 minutes then split them among your plates before eating.

Nutrition: Calories: 222, Fat: 6.7g, Fiber: 1.6g, Carbs: 4.8g, Protein: 34.4g

247. **Peppered Broccoli Chicken**

Preparation Time: 20 minutes
Cooking Time: 30 minutes
Servings: 4
Ingredients:

- 1 tbsp Sage (sliced)
- 1 cup Broccoli florets
- 1 lb. (no bones and skin) Chicken breast
- 3 pieces Garlic cloves
- 1 cup Tomato passata
- What you'll need from the store cupboard:
- Salt and Black pepper to taste
- 2 tbsp. Olive oil

Directions:

1. Put the instant pot on Sauté option, then put the oil and cook it. After that, put the chicken and garlic then heats it for 5 minutes.
2. Put the other ingredients, then cover it and heat it for 25 minutes on high temperature.
3. Release the pressure gradually for 10 minutes then split them among your plates before eating.

Nutrition: Calories: 217, Fat: 10.1g, Fiber: 1.8g, Carbs: 5.9g, Protein: 25.4g

248. **Turkey Coriander Dish**

Preparation Time: 20 minutes
Cooking Time: 20 minutes
Servings: 4
Ingredients:

- half bunch Coriander (sliced)
- 1 cup Chard (sliced)
- 1 piece (no bones and skin) Turkey breast
- 1 and a half cup Coconut cream
- 2 pieces Garlic cloves
- What you'll need from the store cupboard:
- 1 tbsp Melted ghee

Directions:

1. Put the instant pot on Sauté option, then put the ghee and cook it. After that, put the garlic and meat then heat it for 5 minutes.

2. Put the other ingredients, then cover it and heat it for 25 minutes on high temperature.
3. Release the pressure gradually for 10 minutes then split them among your plates before eating.

Nutrition: Calories: 225, Fat: 8.9g, Fiber: 0.2g, Carbs: 0.8g, Protein: 33.5g

249. Peppered Chicken Breast with Basil

Preparation Time: 10 minutes
Cooking Time: 20 minutes
Servings: 4
Ingredients:

- ¼ cup Red bell peppers
- 1 cup Chicken stock
- 2 pieces (no skin and bones) Chicken breasts
- 4 pieces Garlic cloves (crushed)
- 1 and a half tbsp Basil (crushed)
- What you'll need from the store cupboard:
- 1 tbsp Chili powder

Directions:
1. In the instant pot, combine the ingredients then cover them and cook for 25 minutes on high temperature.
2. Release the pressure quickly for 5 minutes then split them among your plates before eating.

Nutrition: Calories: 230, Fat: 12.4g, Fiber: 0.8g, Carbs: 2.7g, Protein: 33.2g

250. Garlic Soy-Glazed Chicken

Preparation Time: 10 minutes
Cooking Time: 25 minutes
Servings: 6
Ingredients:

- 2 pounds' boneless chicken thighs
- What you'll need from the store cupboard:
- Salt and pepper
- 1 tablespoon minced garlic
- ¼ cup soy sauce
- ¾ cup apple cider vinegar

Directions:
1. Season the chicken with salt and pepper, then add it to the Instant Pot, skin-side down.
2. Whisk together the apple cider vinegar, soy sauce, and garlic then add to the pot.
3. Close and lock the lid, then press the Manual button and adjust the timer to 15 minutes.
4. When the timer goes off, let the pressure vent naturally.
5. When the pot has depressurized, open the lid.
6. Remove the chicken to a baking sheet and place under the broiler for 3 to 5 minutes until the skin is crisp.
7. Meanwhile, turn the Instant Pot on to Sauté and cook until the sauce thickens, stirring as needed.
8. Serve the chicken with the sauce spooned over it.

Nutrition: calories 335 fat 23g protein 27.5g carbs 1.5g fiber 0g net carbs 1.5g

251. Coco Turkey in Tomato Pasta

Preparation Time: 15 minutes
Cooking Time: 20 minutes
Servings: 4
Ingredients:

- 1 piece (no bones and skin) Large turkey
- 1 and a half cups Coconut cream
- 2 tbsp Garlic
- 1 tsp Basil
- 2 tbsp Tomato pasta
- What you'll need from the store cupboard:
- Salt and Black pepper to taste
- 1 tbsp Melted ghee

Directions:
1. Put the instant pot on Sauté option, then put the ghee and cook it. After that, put the garlic and meat then heat it for 5 minutes.
2. Put the other ingredients then cover it and heat it for 20 minutes on high temperature.
3. Release the pressure gradually for 10 minutes, then after that split them among your plates before eating.

Nutrition: Calories: 229, Fat: 8.9g, Fiber: 0.2g, Carbs: 1.8g, Protein: 33.6g

252. Cheesy Chicken and Avocado in Tomato Sauce

Preparation Time: 20 minutes
Cooking Time: 10 minutes
Servings: 8
Ingredients:

- 1 cup Shredded cheddar cheese
- 2 Skinless and boneless chicken breast; halved
- 2 Avocados; pitted, peeled and cubed
- 2 cups Tomato passata
- What you'll need from the store cupboard:
- A pinch of salt and black pepper
- 1 tbsp Olive oil

Directions:
1. Press 'Sauté' on the instant pot and pour in the oil. When it is hot, brown the chicken for 5 minutes.
2. Mix in the passata, avocados, salt, and pepper.
3. Spread the cheese over the mix and seal the lid to cook for 12minutes at high pressure.
4. Natural release the pressure for 10 minutes, share into plates and serve.

Nutrition: Calories 198, fat 16.4, carbs 6.6, protein 5.4, fiber 4.6

253. Oregano Flavored Chicken Olives

Preparation Time: 15 minutes
Cooking Time: 15 minutes
Servings: 4
Ingredients:

- 2 pieces (without skin and bones) Chicken breasts
- 2 pieces Eggplants
- 1 tbsp Oregano

- 1 cup Tomato passata
- What you'll need from the store cupboard:
- Salt and Black pepper to taste
- 2 tbsp Olive oil

Directions:
1. In the instant pot mix all the ingredients, then cover them and cook for 20 minutes on high temperature.
2. Release the pressure gradually for 10 minutes then split them among your plates before eating.

Nutrition: Calories: 362, Fat: 16.1, Fiber: 4.4g, Carbs: 5.4g, Protein: 36.4g

254. **Duck with Garlic and Onion Sauce**

Preparation Time: 20 minutes
Cooking Time: 20 minutes
Servings: 4
Ingredients:
- 2 tbsp Coriander
- 2 pieces Spring onions
- 1 lb. (no skin and bones) Duck legs
- 2 pieces Garlic cloves
- 2 tbsp Tomato passata
- What you'll need from the store cupboard:
- 2 tbsp Melted ghee

Directions:
1. Put the instant pot on Sauté option, then put the ghee and cook it. After that, put the spring onions and the other ingredients excluding the tomato passata and the meat then heat it for 5 minutes.
2. Put the meat and cook for 5 minutes.
3. Put the sauce then cover it and heat it for 25 minutes on high temperature.
4. Release the pressure gradually for 10 minutes then split them among your plates before eating.

Nutrition: Calories: 263, Fat: 13.2g, Fiber: 0.2g, Carbs: 1.1g, Protein: 33.5g

255. **Chinese Stuffed Chicken**

Preparation Time: 20 minutes
Cooking Time: 30 minutes
Servings: 8
Ingredients:
- 1 whole chicken
- 10 wolfberries
- 2 red chilies; chopped
- 4 ginger slices
- 1 yam; cubed
- 1 tsp. soy sauce
- 3 tsp. sesame oil
- Salt and white pepper to the taste

Directions:
1. Season chicken with salt, pepper, rub with soy sauce and sesame oil and stuff with wolfberries, yam cubes, chilies and ginger.
2. Place in your air fryer, cook at 400 °F, for 20 minutes and then at 360 °F, for 15 minutes. Carve chicken, divide among plates and serve.

Nutrition: Calories: 320; Fat: 12; Fiber: 17; Carbs: 22; Protein: 12

256. **Chicken and Asparagus**

Preparation Time: 20 minutes
Cooking Time: 10 minutes
Servings: 4
Ingredients:
- 8 chicken wings; halved
- 8 asparagus spears
- 1 tbsp. rosemary; chopped
- 1 tsp. cumin; ground
- Salt and black pepper to the taste

Directions:
1. Pat dry chicken wings, season with salt, pepper, cumin and rosemary, put them in your air fryer's basket and cook at 360 °F, for 20 minutes.
2. Meanwhile; heat up a pan over medium heat, add asparagus, add water to cover, steam for a few minutes; transfer to a bowl filled with ice water, drain and arrange on plates. Add chicken wings on the side and serve.

Nutrition: Calories: 270; Fat: 8; Fiber: 12; Carbs: 24; Protein: 22

257. **Italian Chicken**

Preparation Time: 10 minutes
Cooking Time: 16 minutes
Servings: 4
Ingredients:
- 5 chicken thighs
- 1 tbsp. olive oil
- 1/4 cup parmesan; grated
- 1/2 cup sun dried tomatoes
- 2 garlic cloves; minced
- 1 tbsp. thyme; chopped.
- 1/2 cup heavy cream
- 3/4 cup chicken stock
- 1 tsp. red pepper flakes; crushed
- 2 tbsp. basil; chopped
- Salt and black pepper to the taste

Directions:
1. Season chicken with salt and pepper, rub with half of the oil, place in your preheated air fryer at 350 °F and cook for 4 minutes.
2. Meanwhile; heat up a pan with the rest of the oil over medium high heat, add thyme garlic, pepper flakes, sun dried tomatoes, heavy cream, stock, parmesan, salt and pepper; stir, bring to a simmer, take off heat and transfer to a dish that fits your air fryer.
3. Add chicken thighs on top, introduce in your air fryer and cook at 320 °F, for 12 minutes. Divide among plates and serve with basil sprinkled on top.

Nutrition: Calories: 272; Fat: 9; Fiber: 12; Carbs: 37; Protein: 23

258. **Chinese Chicken Wings**

Preparation Time: 20 minutes
Cooking Time: 10 minutes

Servings: 6
Ingredients:

- 16 chicken wings
- 2 tbsp. honey
- 2 tbsp. soy sauce
- Salt and black pepper to the taste
- 1/4 tsp. white pepper
- 3 tbsp. lime juice

Directions:

1. In a bowl, mix honey with soy sauce, salt, black and white pepper and lime juice, whisk well, add chicken pieces, toss to coat and keep in the fridge for 2 hours.
2. Transfer chicken to your air fryer, cook at 370 °F, for 6 minutes on each side, increase heat to 400 °F and cook for 3 minutes more. Serve hot.

Nutrition: Calories: 372; Fat: 9; Fiber: 10; Carbs: 37; Protein: 24

259. <u>Creamy Chicken, Peas and Rice</u>

Preparation Time: 20 minutes
Cooking Time: 20 minutes
Servings: 4
Ingredients:

- 1 lb. chicken breasts; skinless, boneless and cut into quarters
- 1 cup white rice; already cooked
- 1 cup chicken stock
- 1/4 cup parsley; chopped.
- 2 cups peas; frozen
- 1 ½ cups parmesan; grated
- 1 tbsp. olive oil
- 3 garlic cloves; minced
- 1 yellow onion; chopped
- 1/2 cup white wine
- 1/4 cup heavy cream
- Salt and black pepper to the taste

Directions:

1. Season chicken breasts with salt and pepper, drizzle half of the oil over them, rub well, put in your air fryer's basket and cook them at 360 °F, for 6 minutes.
2. Heat up a pan with the rest of the oil over medium high heat, add garlic, onion, wine, stock, salt, pepper and heavy cream; stir, bring to a simmer and cook for 9 minutes.
3. Transfer chicken breasts to a heat proof dish that fits your air fryer, add peas, rice and cream mix over them, toss, sprinkle parmesan and parsley all over, place in your air fryer and cook at 420 °F, for 10 minutes. Divide among plates and serve hot.

Nutrition: Calories: 313; Fat: 12; Fiber: 14; Carbs: 27; Protein: 44

260. <u>Chicken and Green Onions Sauce</u>

Preparation Time: 10 minutes
Cooking Time: 16 minutes

Servings: 4
Ingredients:

- 10 green onions; roughly chopped.
- 1-inch piece ginger root; chopped
- 4 garlic cloves; minced
- 2 tbsp. fish sauce
- 3 tbsp. soy sauce
- 1 tsp. Chinese five spice
- 10 chicken drumsticks
- 1 cup coconut milk
- 1 tsp. butter; melted
- 1/4 cup cilantro; chopped.
- 1 tbsp. lime juice
- Salt and black pepper to the taste

Directions:

1. In your food processor, mix green onions with ginger, garlic, soy sauce, fish sauce, five spice, salt, pepper, butter and coconut milk and pulse well.
2. In a bowl, mix chicken with green onions mix; toss well, transfer everything to a pan that fits your air fryer and cook at 370 °F, for 16 minutes; shaking the fryer once. Divide among plates, sprinkle cilantro on top, drizzle lime juice and serve with a side salad.

Nutrition: Calories: 321; Fat: 12; Fiber: 12; Carbs: 22; Protein: 20

261. <u>Chicken Cacciatore</u>

Preparation Time: 20 minutes
Cooking Time: 10 minutes
Servings: 4
Ingredients:

- 8 chicken drumsticks; bone-in
- 1/2 cup black olives; pitted and sliced
- 1 bay leaf
- 1 tsp. garlic powder
- 1 yellow onion; chopped
- 28 oz. canned tomatoes and juice; crushed
- 1 tsp. oregano; dried
- Salt and black pepper to the taste

Directions:

1. In a heat proof dish that fits your air fryer, mix chicken with salt, pepper, garlic powder, bay leaf, onion, tomatoes and juice, oregano and olives; toss, introduce in your preheated air fryer and cook at 365 °F, for 20 minutes. Divide among plates and serve.

Nutrition: Calories: 300; Fat: 12; Fiber: 8; Carbs: 20; Protein: 24

262. <u>Herbed Chicken</u>

Preparation Time: 20 minutes
Cooking Time: 50 minutes
Servings: 4
Ingredients:

- 1 whole chicken
- 1 tsp. garlic powder
- 1 tsp. onion powder
- 1/2 tsp. thyme; dried

- 1 tsp. rosemary; dried
- 1 tbsp. lemon juice
- 2 tbsp. olive oil
- Salt and black pepper to the taste

Directions:
1. Season chicken with salt and pepper, rub with thyme, rosemary, garlic powder and onion powder, rub with lemon juice and olive oil and leave aside for 30 minutes.
2. Put chicken in your air fryer and cook at 360 °F, for 20 minutes on each side. Leave chicken aside to cool down, carve and serve.

Nutrition: Calories: 390; Fat: 10; Fiber: 5; Carbs: 22; Protein: 20

263. Air Fried Chicken with Honey and Lemon

Preparation Time: 50 minutes
Cooking Time: 50 minutes
Servings: 4
Ingredients:
- The Stuffing:
- 1 whole chicken, 3 lb
- 2 red and peeled onions
- 2 tbsp olive oil
- 2 apricots
- 1 zucchini
- 1 apple
- 2 cloves finely chopped garlic
- Fresh chopped thyme
- Salt and pepper
- The Marinade:
- 5 oz honey
- juice from 1 lemon
- 2 tbsp olive oil
- Salt and pepper

Directions:
1. For the stuffing, chop all ingredients into tiny pieces. Transfer to a large bowl and add the olive oil. Season with salt and black pepper. Fill the cavity of the chicken with the stuffing, without packing it tightly.
2. Place the chicken in the Air Fryer and cook for 35 minutes at 340 F. Warm the honey and the lemon juice in a large pan; season with salt and pepper. Reduce the temperature of the Air Fryer to 320 F.
3. Brush the chicken with some of the honey-lemon marinade and return it to the fryer. Cook for another 70 minutes; brush the chicken every 20-25 minutes with the marinade. Garnish with parsley, and serve with potatoes.

Nutrition: Calories: 342; Carbs: 68g; Fat: 28g; Protein: 33g

264. 400: Spicy Honey Orange Chicken

Preparation Time: 10 minutes
Cooking Time: 10 minutes
Servings: 4
Ingredients:

- 1 ½ pounds chicken breast, washed and sliced
- Parsley to taste
- 1 cup coconut, shredded
- ¾ cup breadcrumbs
- 2 whole eggs, beaten
- ½ cup flour
- ½ tsp pepper
- Salt to taste
- ½ cup orange marmalade
- 1 tbsp red pepper flakes
- ¼ cup honey
- 3 tbsp dijon mustard

Directions:
1. Preheat your Air Fryer to 400 F. In a mixing bowl, combine coconut, flour, salt, parsley and pepper. In another bowl, add the beaten eggs. Place breadcrumbs in a third bowl. Dredge chicken in egg mix, flour and finally in the breadcrumbs. Place the chicken in the Air Fryer cooking basket and bake for 15 minutes.
2. In a separate bowl, mix honey, orange marmalade, mustard and pepper flakes. Cover chicken with marmalade mixture and fry for 5 more minutes. Enjoy!

Nutrition: Calories: 246; Carbs: 21g; Fat: 6g; Protein: 25g

265. Crunchy Chicken Fingers

Preparation Time: 4 minutes
Cooking Time: 4 minutes
Servings: 2
Ingredients:
- 2 medium-sized chicken breasts, cut in stripes
- 3 tbsp parmesan cheese
- ¼ tbsp fresh chives, chopped
- ⅓ cup breadcrumbs
- 1 egg white
- 2 tbsp plum sauce, optional
- ½ tbsp fresh thyme, chopped
- ½ tbsp black pepper
- 1 tbsp water

Directions:
1. Preheat the Air Fryer to 360 F. Mix the chives, parmesan, thyme, pepper and breadcrumbs. In another bowl, whisk the egg white and mix with the water. Dip the chicken strips into the egg mixture and the breadcrumb mixture. Place the strips in the air fryer basket and cook for 10 minutes. Serve with plum sauce.

Nutrition: Calories: 253; Carbs: 31g; Fat: 18g; Protein: 28g

266. Mustard and Maple Turkey Breast

Preparation Time: 20 minutes
Cooking Time: 1 hr
Servings: 6
Ingredients:
- 5 lb of whole turkey breast
- ¼ cup maple syrup

- 2 tbsp dijon mustard
- ½ tbsp smoked paprika
- 1 tbsp thyme
- 2 tbsp olive oil
- ½ tbsp sage
- ½ tbsp salt and black pepper
- 1 tbsp butter, melted

Directions:
1. Preheat the Air fryer to 350 F and brush the turkey with the olive oil. Combine all herbs and seasoning, in a small bowl, and rub the turkey with the mixture. Air fry the turkey for 25 minutes. Flip the turkey on its side and continue to cook for 12 more minutes.
2. Now, turn on the opposite side, and again, cook for an additional 12 minutes. Whisk the butter, maple and mustard together in a small bowl. When done, brush the glaze all over the turkey. Return to the air fryer and cook for 5 more minutes, until nice and crispy.

Nutrition: Calories: 529; Carbs: 77g; Fat: 20g; Protein: 13g

267. Chicken Breasts with Tarragon

Preparation Time: 20 minutes
Cooking Time: 15 minutes
Servings: 3
Ingredients:
- 1 boneless and skinless chicken breast
- ½ tbsp butter
- ¼ tbsp kosher salt
- ¼ cup dried tarragon
- ¼ tbsp black and fresh ground pepper

Directions:
1. Preheat the Air Fryer to 380 F and place each chicken breast on a 12x12 inches foil wrap. Top the chicken with tarragon and butter; season with salt and pepper to taste. Wrap the foil around the chicken breast in a loose way to create a flow of air. Cook the in the Air Fryer for 15 minutes. Carefully unwrap the chicken and serve.

Nutrition: Calories: 493; Carbs: 36.5g; Fat: 11g; Protein: 57.5g

268. Chicken with Cashew Nuts

Preparation Time: 20 minutes
Cooking Time: 30 minutes
Servings: 4
Ingredients:
- 1 lb chicken cubes
- 2 tbsp soy sauce
- 1 tbsp corn flour
- 2 ½ onion cubes
- 1 carrot, chopped
- ⅓ cup cashew nuts, fried
- 1 capsicum, cut
- 2 tbsp garlic, crushed
- Salt and white pepper

Directions:

1. Marinate the chicken cubes with ½ tbsp of white pepper, ½ tsp salt, 2 tbsp soya sauce, and add 1 tbsp corn flour.
2. Set aside for 25 minutes. Preheat the Air Fryer to 380 F and transfer the marinated chicken. Add the garlic, the onion, the capsicum, and the carrot; fry for 5-6 minutes. Roll it in the cashew nuts before serving.

Nutrition: Calories: 425; Carbs: 25g; Fat: 35g; Protein: 53g

269. Chicken Cabbage Curry

Preparation Time: 20 minutes
Cooking Time: 30 minutes
Servings: 4
Ingredients:
- 1 kg of boneless chicken, cut into small pieces
- 2 cans of coconut milk
- 3 tablespoons of curry paste
- 1 small onion, diced
- 1 medium red bell pepper
- 1 medium green bell pepper
- 1/2 head of a big cabbage

Directions:
1. Dissolve the curry paste into the coconut milk and stir well. Pour into the Instant Pot.
2. Add the chicken to the coconut curry mixture.
3. Chop both peppers into cubes and add to the pot.
4. Add the onion.
5. Cut the cabbage into slices and add to the pot. Make sure all the ingredients are coated with coconut milk.
6. Put the lid on, seal and cook on Low for 30 minutes.
7. When it's cooked, open carefully and serve immediately.

Nutrition: Calories 301 Fat 27.2 g Carbohydrates 13.6 g Sugar 6 g Protein 4.9 g Cholesterol 33 mg

270. Chicken Salad

Preparation Time: 20 minutes
Cooking Time: 30 minutes
Servings: 6
Ingredients:
- 1 kg chicken breast
- 125 ml chicken broth
- 1 teaspoon salt
- ½ teaspoon black pepper

Directions:
1. Add all of the ingredients to the Instant Pot.
2. Secure the lid, close the pressure valve and cook for 20 minutes at High pressure.
3. Quick release pressure.
4. Shred the chicken. Store in an air-tight container with the liquid to help keep the meat moist.

Nutrition: Calories 356 Fat 27.2 g Carbohydrates 13.6 g Sugar 3 g Protein 4.9 g Cholesterol 5 mg

271. Lemony Chicken Casserole

Preparation Time: 20 minutes
Cooking Time: 30 minutes
Servings: 4

Ingredients:

- 2 tablespoons olive oil
- 200 ml chicken broth
- Juice of one lemon
- 1 kg chicken thighs
- 2-3 tablespoons Dijon mustard
- 2 tablespoons Mediterranean seasoning
- 800 gr red potatoes, quartered
- Salt and pepper to taste

Directions:

1. Add oil to Instant Pot.
2. Season the chicken thighs with salt and pepper and add to Instant Pot.
3. Combine chicken broth, lemon juice, and Dijon mustard, and pour over chicken.
4. Add quartered potatoes and seasoning
5. Place lid on Instant Pot and cook on Manual for 15 minutes.
6. Quick Release when the pot beeps.

Nutrition: Calories 301 Fat 27.2 g Carbohydrates 13.6 g Sugar 6 g Protein 4.9 g Cholesterol 33 mg

272. **Chicken Tikka Masala**

Preparation Time: 20 minutes
Cooking Time: 10 minutes
Servings: 4
Ingredients:

- 2 tablespoons olive oil
- 1 small onion, diced
- 3 cloves garlic, minced
- 1 (2-inch) piece fresh ginger, peeled and grated
- 1/2 cup chicken broth,
- 1 1/2 tablespoons garam masala
- 1 teaspoon paprika
- 1/2 teaspoon ground turmeric
- 1/2 teaspoon salt
- 1/4 teaspoon cayenne pepper
- 750 gr boneless, skinless chicken meat, cut into small pieces
- 450 g can tomatoes, juices included
- 1/2 cup coconut milk
- Fresh cilantro, chopped

Directions:

1. Set the cooker to the Sauté. Add the oil, and when it's hot, add the onion and sauté until softened, about 3 minutes. Add the garlic and ginger and cook until soft.
2. Add half of the chicken broth. Cook for couple of minutes, stirring all the time, add the garam masala, paprika, turmeric, salt, and cayenne pepper, and stir to combine.
3. Add the chicken and the remaining chicken broth and the tomatoes.
4. Close and lock the lid. Pressure-cook for 10 minutes at High pressure. When it's cooked, do a quick release of the pressure.
5. Stir the coconut milk into the sauce.

6. Serving suggestion: Serve on a bed of cauliflower "rice", or boiled potatoes.

Nutrition: Calories 245 Fat 25 g Carbohydrates 12.6 g Sugar 4 g Protein 5 g Cholesterol 35 mg

273. **Juicy Whole Chicken**

Preparation Time: 10 minutes
Cooking Time: 30 minutes
Servings: 6
Ingredients:

- 2 tbsp olive oil
- 300 ml chicken broth
- 3 red potatoes
- 1 chicken, whole
- Spices of your choice, eg thyme, oregano, salt, garlic salt

Directions:

1. Put your Instant Pot on Saute, Low Setting.
2. Add olive oil and when it's hot, add chicken to the pot and lightly cook for about 2 minutes. Repeat with the other side. Turn off by pressing Cancel.
3. Remove browned meat from Instant Pot and add chicken broth, potatoes, and the chicken (whole or in pieces). Chicken should be on top of the potatoes.
4. Close lid, make sure steam valve is secure, and set to Poultry, normal setting, for 25 minutes. When it's cooked, do a quick release

Nutrition: Calories 301 Fat 27.2 g Carbohydrates 13.6 g Sugar 6 g Protein 4.9 g Cholesterol 33 mg

274. **Spicy Lime Chicken Breasts**

Preparation Time: 20 minutes
Cooking Time: 20 minutes
Servings: 5
Ingredients:

- 2 tablespoons zest lime
- 2 tablespoons honey
- 1 tablespoon lime juice
- 3 teaspoons mince garlic
- Salt and pepper to taste
- ½ teaspoon chili powder
- 1 ½ teaspoon paprika
- 1 teaspoon allspice, ground
- 1.5 kg chicken

Directions:

1. In a bowl, combine lime zest, honey, lime juice, garlic, pepper, sea salt, chili powder, paprika and allspice. Coat chicken in marinade.
2. Pour broth in Instant Pot, then add chicken.
3. Lock lid into place and seal steam nozzle.
4. Cook on High pressure for 15 minutes.
5. Naturally release pressure for 5 minutes then release any remaining pressure.
6. Open the Pot carefully, and serve.

Nutrition: Calories 325 Fat 27.2 g Carbohydrates 13.6 g Sugar 7 g Protein 5 g Cholesterol 36 mg

275. **Whole Roasted Chicken**

Preparation Time: 20 minutes
Cooking Time: 10 minutes

Servings: 6

Ingredients:

- 1 whole chicken (about 2 kg)
- 1 tablespoon chopped fresh rosemary
- 1 1/2-2 tablespoons olive oil, plus a bit more for drizzling in pan
- 4-6 cloves garlic
- 1/2 teaspoon paprika
- Salt and pepper to taste
- Zest from 1 lemon
- 1 cup chicken broth
- 1 large onion, quartered

Directions:

1. Rinse the chicken with cold water and pat dry with paper towels. Place in baking pan and set aside.
2. Preheat Instant Pot and go to Saute mode.
3. In a small bowl combine rosemary, olive oil, garlic, paprika, salt, pepper, and lemon zest. After removing the zest, cut lemon in half and stuff in cavity of chicken. Spread spice mixture all over the chicken, spreading evenly. Drizzle some olive oil in your hot pan and place chicken breast-side down into pot. Leave for 3-4 minutes, until golden brown. Flip chicken over and bake the other side.
4. Remove chicken from pan and set onto the baking dish where it was before. Add broth to pan. Place onion on bottom of pan, place chicken on top (breast-side up) and secure lid.
5. Cook on High pressure for 6 minutes per pound. When it's cooked, wait for 10 minutes before releasing steam. Remove chicken and wait for at least 5 minutes before slicing.

Nutrition: Calories 301 Fat 27.2 g Carbohydrates 13.6 g Sugar 6 g Protein 4.9 g Cholesterol 33 mg

276. Italian Style Chicken Breast

Preparation Time: 20 minutes
Cooking Time: 15 minutes
Servings: 3

Ingredients:

- 1 tablespoon olive oil
- 3 boneless, skinless chicken breasts
- 1/4 teaspoon garlic powder and regular salt per breast
- dash black pepper
- 1/8 teaspoon dried oregano
- 1/8 teaspoon dried basil
- 250 ml water

Directions:

1. Set the Instant Pot to Saute, and add oil to the pot.
2. Season one side of the chicken breasts and once the oil is hot, carefully add the chicken breasts, seasoned side down, to the pot.
3. In the meantime, season the second side.
4. Cook about 3 to 4 minutes on each side, and remove from pot with the tongs.
5. Add 250 ml water to the pot, plus the trivet.
6. Place the chicken on the trivet.

7. Lock the lid, and cook on manual High for 5 minutes.
8. Allow the chicken to naturally release for a few minutes, and then quick release the rest.
9. Remove from the pot and wait for at least 5 minutes before slicing.

Nutrition: Calories 202 Fat 29 g Carbohydrates 13.6 g Sugar 6 g Protein 4.9 g Cholesterol 33 mg

277. Rosemary Lemon Chicken

Preparation Time: 20 minutes
Cooking Time: 14 minutes
Servings: 4

Ingredients:

- 1 kg chicken breast halves
- 1 lemon, peeled and sliced into rounds
- 1/2 orange, peeled and sliced into rounds, or to taste
- 3 cloves roasted garlic, or to taste
- salt and ground black pepper to taste
- 1 1/2 tablespoons olive oil, or to taste
- 1 1/2 teaspoons agave syrup, or to taste (optional)
- 1/4 cup water
- 2 sprigs fresh rosemary, stemmed, or to taste

Directions:

1. Place chicken in the Instant Pot. Add lemon, orange, and garlic; season with salt and pepper. Drizzle olive oil and agave syrup (if using) on top. Add water and rosemary. Put the lid on the cooker and Lock in place.
2. Select the "Meat" and "Stew" settings for High pressure, and cook for 14 minutes. Allow pressure to release naturally, about 20 minutes.

Nutrition: Calories 325 Fat 5 g Carbohydrates 20 g Sugar 2 g Protein 10 g Cholesterol 33 mg

278. Spicy Chicken Drumsticks

Preparation Time: 20 minutes
Cooking Time: 10 minutes
Servings: 6

Ingredients:

- 1/2 cup ketchup
- 1/4 cup dark brown sugar
- 1/4 cup red wine vinegar
- 3 tablespoon soy sauce
- 1 tablespoon chicken seasoning
- Salt to taste
- 6 chicken drumsticks

Directions:

1. Combine ketchup, brown sugar, red wine vinegar, soy sauce, seasoning, and salt in the Instant Pot. Add chicken pieces and stir to coat.
2. Close Instant Pot Lid, and make sure steam release handle is in the 'Sealing' position.
3. Cook on 'Manual' (or 'Pressure Cook') for 12 minutes.
4. Do a quick release of pressure and carefully open the Instant Pot.
5. Remove chicken pieces and set aside.

6. Press 'Saute' and cook the sauce thickened, about 5 to 7 minutes.

Nutrition: Calories 145 Fat 28 g Carbohydrates 13.6 g Sugar 2 g Protein 4.9 g Cholesterol 45 mg

279. Ginger Flavored Chicken

Preparation Time: 20 minutes
Cooking Time: 15 minutes
Servings: 6
Ingredients

- 1 kg boneless, skinless chicken breasts (frozen OR thawed)
- 6 tablespoons soy sauce
- 3 tablespoons rice vinegar
- 1/2 tablespoon honey
- 3 tablespoons water, broth, or orange juice
- 2 tablespoons chopped fresh ginger
- 6 cloves garlic, minced
- 3 teaspoons corn starch

Directions:
1. Place chicken breasts in Instant Pot.
2. In a small mixing bowl, whisk together: vinegar, soy sauce, honey, water, ginger and garlic. Pour mixture over chicken and coat evenly.
3. Secure lid on Instant Pot and cook at High pressure for 15 minutes. When the meat is cooked, release steam.
4. Remove chicken breasts and place on a cutting board. Bring remaining sauce in pan up to a simmer (use the Saute feature on an electric cooker). Combine cornstarch with 3 teaspoons cold water and then pour mixture into pan. Simmer until sauce is thickened and the turn off heat.
5. Shred chicken and return to pot with sauce.

Nutrition: Calories 313 Fat 25.6 g Carbohydrates 15.6 g Sugar 7 g Protein 8 g Cholesterol 36 mg

280. Buffalo Chicken

Preparation Time: 20 minutes
Cooking Time: 30 minutes
Servings: 8
Ingredients:

- 2 celery stalks, diced
- 1 medium-sized onion, chopped
- 100 ml buffalo wing sauce
- 100 ml chicken broth
- 21 kg chicken breasts, frozen

Directions:
1. Add the celery, onions, wing sauce, chicken broth and chicken to the Instant Pot. Cook frozen chicken on high pressure for 20 minutes. Turn the pressure valve to "Vent" to release all of the pressure.
2. Remove the chicken breasts from the pot, and shred.
3. You can remove most of the liquid from the pot, or not.

Nutrition: Calories: 197 Fat: 8g Carbohydrates: 16g Protein: 14g

281. Breaded Chicken with Seed Chips

Preparation time: 10 minutes
Cooking time: 40 minutes
Servings: 4
Ingredients:

- 12 chicken breast fillets
- Salt
- 2 eggs
- 1 small bag of seed chips
- Breadcrumbs
- Extra virgin olive oil

Directions:
1. Put salt to chicken fillets.
2. Crush the seed chips and when we have them fine, bind with the breadcrumbs.
3. Beat the two eggs.
4. Pass the chicken breast fillets through the beaten egg and then through the seed chips that you have tied with the breadcrumbs.
5. When you have them all breaded, paint with a brush of extra virgin olive oil.
6. Place the fillets in the basket of the air fryer without being piled up.
7. Select 170 degrees, 20 minutes.
8. Take out and put another batch, repeat temperature and time. So, until you use up all the steaks.

Nutrition: Calories: 242 Fat: 13g Carbohydrates: 13.5g Protein: 18g Sugar: 0g Cholesterol: 42mg

282. Salted Biscuit Pie Turkey Chops

Preparation time: 5 minutes
Cooking time: 20 minutes
Servings: 4
Ingredients:

- 8 large turkey chops
- 300 gr of crackers
- 2 eggs
- Extra virgin olive oil
- Salt
- Ground pepper

Direction:
1. Put the turkey chops on the worktable, and salt and pepper.
2. Beat the eggs in a bowl.
3. Crush the cookies in the Thermo mix with a few turbo strokes until they are made grit, or you can crush them with the blender.
4. Put the cookies in a bowl.
5. Pass the chops through the beaten egg and then passed them through the crushed cookies. Press well so that the empanada is perfect.
6. Paint the empanada with a silicone brush and extra virgin olive oil.
7. Put the chops in the basket of the air fryer, not all will enter. They will be done in batches.
8. Select 200 degrees, 15 minutes.
9. When you have all the chops made, serve.

Nutrition: Calories: 126 Fat: 6g Carbohydrates 0g Protein: 18g Sugar: 0g

283. Lemon Chicken with Basil

Preparation time: 10 minutes
Cooking time: 1h
Servings: 4
Ingredients:

- 1kg chopped chicken
- 1 or 2 lemons
- Basil, salt, and ground pepper
- Extra virgin olive oil

Direction:

1. Put the chicken in a bowl with a jet of extra virgin olive oil.
2. Put salt, pepper, and basil.
3. Bind well and let stand for at least 30 minutes stirring occasionally.
4. Put the pieces of chicken in the air fryer basket and take the air fryer
5. Select 30 minutes.
6. Occasionally remove.
7. Take out and put another batch.
8. Do the same operation.

Nutrition: Calories: 126 Fat: 6g Carbohydrates 0g Protein: 18g Sugar: 0g

284. Fried Chicken Tamari and Mustard

Preparation time: 15 minutes
Cooking time: 1h 20 minutes
Servings: 4
Ingredients:

- 1kg of very small chopped chicken
- Tamari Sauce
- Original mustard
- Ground pepper
- 1 lemon
- Flour
- Extra virgin olive oil

Directions:

1. Put the chicken in a bowl, you can put the chicken with or without the skin, to everyone's taste.
2. Add a generous stream of tamari, one or two tablespoons of mustard, a little ground pepper and a splash of lemon juice.
3. Link everything very well and let macerate an hour.
4. Pass the chicken pieces for flour and place in the air fryer basket.
5. Put 20 minutes at 200 degrees. At half time, move the chicken from the basket.
6. Do not crush the chicken, it is preferable to make two or three batches of chicken to pile up and do not fry the pieces well.

Nutrition: Calories: 100 Fat: 6g Carbohydrates 0g Protein: 18g Sugar: 0g

285. Breaded Chicken Fillets

Preparation time: 10 minutes
Cooking time: 25 minutes
Servings: 4

Ingredients:

- 3 small chicken breasts or 2 large chicken breasts
- Salt
- Ground pepper
- 3 garlic cloves
- 1 lemon
- Beaten eggs
- Breadcrumbs
- Extra virgin olive oil

Direction:

1. Cut the breasts into fillets.
2. Put in a bowl and add the lemon juice, chopped garlic cloves and pepper.
3. Flirt well and leave 10 minutes.
4. Beat the eggs and put breadcrumbs on another plate.
5. Pass the chicken breast fillets through the beaten egg and the breadcrumbs.
6. When you have them all breaded, start to fry.
7. Paint the breaded breasts with a silicone brush and extra virgin olive oil.
8. Place a batch of fillets in the basket of the air fryer and select 10 minutes 180 degrees.
9. Turn around and leave another 5 minutes at 180 degrees.

Nutrition: Calories: 120 Fat: 6g Carbohydrates 0g Protein: 18g Sugar: 0g

286. Dry Rub Chicken Wings

Preparation time: 5 minutes
Cooking time: 30 minutes
Servings: 4
Ingredients:

- 9g garlic powder
- 1 cube of chicken broth, reduced sodium
- 5g of salt
- 3g black pepper
- 1g smoked paprika
- 1g cayenne pepper
- 3g Old Bay seasoning, sodium free
- 3g onion powder
- 1g dried oregano
- 453g chicken wings
- Nonstick Spray Oil
- Ranch sauce, to serve

Direction:

1. Preheat the air fryer. Set the temperature to 180 °C.
2. Put ingredients in a bowl and mix well.
3. Season the chicken wings with half the seasoning mixture and sprinkle abundantly with oil spray.
4. Place the chicken wings in the preheated air fryer.
5. Select Chicken, set the timer to 30 minutes.
6. Shake the baskets halfway through cooking.

Nutrition: Calories: 120 Fat: 6g Carbohydrates 0g Protein: 18g Sugar: 0g

287. Chicken Soup

Preparation Time: 20 minutes
Cooking Time: 30 minutes

Servings: 6
Ingredients:

- 4 lbs Chicken, cut into pieces
- 5 carrots, sliced thick
- 8 cups of water
- 2 celery stalks, sliced 1 inch thick
- 2 large onions, sliced

Directions:

1. In a large pot add chicken, water, and salt. Bring to boil.
2. Add celery and onion in the pot and stir well.
3. Turn heat to medium-low and simmer for 30 minutes.
4. Add carrots and cover pot with a lid and simmer for 40 minutes.
5. Remove Chicken from the pot and remove bones and cut Chicken into bite-size pieces.
6. Return chicken into the pot and stir well.
7. Serve and enjoy.

Nutrition: Calories: 89 Fat: 6.33g Carbohydrates: 0g Protein: 7.56g Sugar: 0g Cholesterol: 0mg

288. Ginger Chili Broccoli

Preparation Time: 10 minutes
Cooking Time: 15 minutes
Servings: 5
Ingredients:

- 8 cups broccoli florets
- 1/2 cup olive oil
- 2 fresh lime juice
- 2 tbsp fresh ginger, grated
- 2 tsp chili pepper, chopped

Directions:

1. Add broccoli florets into the steamer and steam for 8 minutes.
2. Meanwhile, for dressing in a small bowl, combine limejuice, oil, ginger, and chili pepper.
3. Add steamed broccoli in a large bowl then pour dressing over broccoli. Toss well.

Nutrition: Calories 239 Fat 20.8 g Carbohydrates 13.7 g Sugar 3 g Protein 4.5 g Cholesterol 0 mg

289. Chicken Wings with Garlic Parmesan

Preparation time: 5 minutes.
Cooking time: 25 minutes
Servings: 3
Ingredients:

- 25g cornstarch
- 20g grated Parmesan cheese
- 9g garlic powder
- Salt and pepper to taste
- 680g chicken wings
- Nonstick Spray Oil

Direction:

1. Select Preheat, set the temperature to 200 °C and press Start / Pause.
2. Combine corn starch, Parmesan, garlic powder, salt, and pepper in a bowl.

3. Mix the chicken wings in the seasoning and dip until well coated.
4. Spray the baskets and the air fryer with oil spray and add the wings, sprinkling the tops of the wings as well.
5. Select Chicken and press Start/Pause. Be sure to shake the baskets in the middle of cooking.
6. Sprinkle with what's left of the Parmesan mix and serve.

Nutrition: Calories: 204 Fat: 15g Carbohydrates: 1g Proteins: 12g Sugar: 0g Cholesterol: 63mg

290. Jerk Style Chicken Wings

Preparation time: 5 minutes.
Cooking time: 25 minutes.
Servings: 2-3
Ingredients:

- 1g ground thyme
- 1g dried rosemary
- 2g allspice
- 4g ground ginger
- 3 g garlic powder
- 2g onion powder
- 1g of cinnamon
- 2g of paprika
- 2g chili powder
- 1g nutmeg
- Salt to taste
- 30 ml of vegetable oil
- 0.5 - 1 kg of chicken wings
- 1 lime, juice

Directions:

1. Select Preheat, set the temperature to 200°C and press Start/Pause.
2. Combine all spices and oil in a bowl to create a marinade.
3. Mix the chicken wings in the marinade until they are well covered.
4. Place the chicken wings in the preheated air fryer.
5. Select Chicken and press Start/Pause. Be sure to shake the baskets in the middle of cooking.
6. Remove the wings and place them on a serving plate.
7. Squeeze fresh lemon juice over the wings and serve.

Nutrition: Calories: 240 Fat: 15g Carbohydrate: 5g Protein: 19g Sugars: 4g Cholesterol: 60mg

291. Tasty Chicken Tenders

Preparation time: 5 minutes.
Cooking time: 25 minutes.
Servings: 4
Ingredients:

- 1 ½ lbs chicken tenders
- 1 tbsp. extra virgin olive oil
- 1 tsp. rotisserie chicken seasoning
- 2 tbsp. BBQ sauce

Directions:

1. Add all ingredients except oil in a zip-lock bag.
2. Seal bag and place in the refrigerator for 2-3 hours.

3. Heat oil in a large pan over medium heat.
4. Cook marinated chicken tenders in a pan until lightly brown and cooked.

Nutrition: Calories 365 Fat 16.1 g, Carbohydrates 2.8 g, Sugar 2 g, Protein 49.2 g, Cholesterol 151 mg

292. Chicken Skewers with Yogurt

Preparation time: 4h 10 minutes.
Cooking time: 10 minutes.
Servings: 2-4
Ingredients:

- 123g of plain whole milk Greek yogurt
- 20 ml of olive oil
- 2g of paprika
- 1g cumin
- 1g crushed red pepper
- 1 lemon, juice and zest of the peel
- 5g of salt
- 1g freshly ground black pepper
- 4 cloves garlic, minced
- 454g chicken thighs, boneless, skinless, cut into 38 mm pieces
- 2 wooden skewers, cut in half
- Nonstick Spray Oil

Direction:

1. Mix the yogurt, olive oil, paprika, cumin, red paprika, lemon juice, lemon zest, salt, pepper, and garlic in a large bowl.
2. Add the chicken to the marinade and marinate in the fridge for at least 4 hours.
3. Select Preheat and press Start/Pause.
4. Cut the marinated chicken thighs into 38 mm pieces and spread them on skewers.
5. Place the skewers in the preheated air fryer.

6. Cook at 200°C for 10 minutes.

Nutrition: Calories: 113 Fat: 3.4 Carbohydrates: 0g Protein: 20.6g

293. Fried Lemon Chicken

Preparation time: 5 minutes.
Cooking time: 20 minutes.
Servings: 6
Ingredients:

- 6 chicken thighs
- 2 tbsp. olive oil
- 2 tbsp. lemon juice
- 1 tbsp. Italian herbal seasoning mix
- 1 tsp. Celtic sea salt
- 1 tsp. ground fresh pepper
- 1 lemon, thinly slice

Directions:

1. Add all ingredients, except sliced lemon, to bowl or bag, stir to cover chicken.
2. Let marinate for 30 minutes overnight.
3. Remove the chicken and let the excess oil drip (it does not need to dry out, just do not drip with tons of excess oil).
4. Arrange the chicken thighs and the lemon slices in the fryer basket, being careful not to push the chicken thighs too close to each other.
5. Set the fryer to 200 degrees and cook for 10 minutes.
6. Remove the basket from the fryer and turn the chicken thighs to the other side.
7. Cook again at 200 for another 10 minutes.

Nutrition: Calories: 215 Fat: 13g Carbohydrates: 1g Protein: 2 Sugar: 1g Cholesterol: 130mg

VEGETABLE RECIPES

294. Dried Fruit Squash

Preparation time: 15 minutes
Cooking time: 40 minutes
Servings: 4
Ingredients:

- ¼ cup water
- 1 medium butternut squash, halved and seeded
- ½ tablespoon olive oil
- ½ tablespoon balsamic vinegar
- Salt and ground black pepper, to taste
- 4 large dates, pitted and chopped
- 4 fresh figs, chopped
- 3 tablespoons pistachios, chopped
- 2 tablespoons pumpkin seeds

Directions:

1. Preheat the oven to 375°F.
2. Place the water in the bottom of a baking dish.
3. Arrange the squash halves in a large baking dish, hollow-side up, and drizzle with oil and vinegar.
4. Sprinkle with salt and black pepper.
5. Spread the dates, figs, and pistachios on top.
6. Bake for about 40 minutes, or until squash becomes tender.
7. Serve hot with the garnishing of pumpkin seeds.

Nutrition: Calories 227 Total Fat 5.5 g Saturated Fat 0.8 g Cholesterol 0 mg Sodium 66 mg Total Carbs 46.4 g Fiber 7.5 g Sugar 19.6 g Protein 5 g

295. Banana Curry

Preparation time: 15 minutes
Cooking time: 15 minutes
Servings: 3
Ingredients:

- 2 tablespoons olive
- 2 yellow onions, chopped
- 8 garlic cloves, minced
- 2 tablespoons curry powder
- 1 tablespoon ground ginger
- 1 tablespoon ground cumin
- 1 teaspoon ground turmeric
- 1 teaspoon ground cinnamon
- 1 teaspoon red chili powder
- Salt and ground black pepper, to taste
- 2/3 cup soy yogurt
- 1 cup tomato puree
- 2 bananas, peeled and sliced
- 3 tomatoes, chopped finely
- ¼ cup unsweetened coconut flakes

Directions:

1. In a large pan, heat the oil over medium heat and sauté onion for about 4–5 minutes.
2. Add the garlic, curry powder, and spices, and sauté for about 1 minute.
3. Add the soy yogurt and tomato sauce and bring to a gentle boil.
4. Stir in the bananas and simmer for about 3 minutes.
5. Stir in the tomatoes and simmer for about 1–2 minutes.
6. Stir in the coconut flakes and immediately remove from the heat.
7. Serve hot.

Nutrition: Calories 382 Total Fat 18.2 g Saturated Fat 6.6 g Cholesterol 0 mg Sodium 108 mg Total Carbs 53.4 g Fiber 11.3 g Sugar 24.8 g Protein 9 g

296. Mushroom Curry

Preparation time: 15 minutes
Cooking time: 20 minutes
Servings: 3
Ingredients:

- 2 cups tomatoes, chopped
- 1 green chili, chopped
- 1 teaspoon fresh ginger, chopped
- ¼ cup cashews
- 2 tablespoons canola oil
- ½ teaspoon cumin seeds
- ¼ teaspoon ground coriander
- ¼ teaspoon ground turmeric
- ¼ teaspoon red chili powder
- 1½ cups fresh shiitake mushrooms, sliced
- 1½ cups fresh button mushrooms, sliced
- 1 cup frozen corn kernels
- 1¼ cups water
- ¼ cup unsweetened coconut milk
- Salt and ground black pepper, to taste

Directions:

1. In a food processor, add the tomatoes, green chili, ginger, and cashews, and pulse until a smooth paste forms.
2. In a pan, heat the oil over medium heat and sauté the cumin seeds for about 1 minute.
3. Add the spices and sauté for about 1 minute.
4. Add the tomato paste and cook for about 5 minutes.
5. Stir in the mushrooms, corn, water, and coconut milk, and bring to a boil.
6. Cook for about 10–12 minutes, stirring occasionally.
7. Season with salt and black pepper and remove from the heat.
8. Serve hot.

Nutrition: Calories 311 Total Fat 20.4 g Saturated Fat 6.1 g Cholesterol 0 mg Sodium 244 mg Total Carbs 32g Fiber 5.6 g Sugar 9 g Protein 8 g

297. 3-Veggie Combo

Preparation time: 15 minutes
Cooking time: 25 minutes
Servings: 4
Ingredients:

- 1 tablespoon olive oil
- 1 small yellow onion, chopped

- 1 teaspoon fresh thyme, chopped
- 1 garlic clove, minced
- 8 ounces' fresh button mushroom, sliced
- 1 pound Brussels sprouts
- 3 cups fresh spinach
- 4 tablespoons walnuts
- Salt and ground black pepper, to taste

Directions:
1. In a large skillet, heat the oil over medium heat and sauté the onion for about 3–4 minutes.
2. Add the thyme and garlic and sauté for about 1 minute.
3. Add the mushrooms and cook for about 15 minutes, or until caramelized.
4. Add the Brussels sprouts and cook for about 2–3 minutes.
5. Stir in the spinach and cook for about 3–4 minutes.
6. Stir in the walnuts, salt, and black pepper, and remove from the heat.
7. Serve hot.

Nutrition: Calories 153 Total Fat 8.8 g Saturated Fat 0.9 g Cholesterol 0 mg Sodium 94 mg Total Carbs 15.8 g Fiber 6.3 g Sugar 4.4 g Protein 8.5 g

298. Beet Soup

Preparation time: 10 minutes
Cooking time: 5 minutes
Servings: 2
Ingredients:

- 2 cups coconut yogurt
- 4 teaspoons fresh lemon juice
- 2 cups beets, trimmed, peeled, and chopped
- 2 tablespoons fresh dill
- Salt, to taste
- 1 tablespoon pumpkin seeds
- 2 tablespoons coconut cream
- 1 tablespoon fresh chives, minced

Directions:
1. In a high-speed blender, add all ingredients and pulse until smooth.
2. Transfer the soup into a pan over medium heat and cook for about 3–5 minutes or until heated through.
3. Serve immediately with the garnishing of chives and coconut cream.

Nutrition: Calories 230 Total Fat 8 g Saturated Fat 5.8 g Cholesterol 0 mg Sodium 218 mg Total Carbs 33.5 g Fiber 4.2 g Sugar 27.5 g Protein 8 g

299. Veggie Stew

Preparation time: 15 minutes
Cooking time: 30 minutes
Servings: 3
Ingredients:

- 2 tablespoons olive oil
- 1 large onion, chopped
- 2 garlic cloves, minced
- ¼ teaspoon fresh ginger, grated finely
- 1 teaspoon ground cumin

- 1 teaspoon cayenne pepper
- Salt and ground black pepper, to taste
- 2 cups homemade vegetable broth
- 1½ cups small broccoli florets
- 1½ cups small cauliflower florets
- 1 tablespoon fresh lemon juice
- 1 cup cashews
- 1 teaspoon fresh lemon zest, grated finely

Directions:
1. In a large soup pan, heat oil over medium heat and sauté the onion for about 3–4 minutes.
2. Add the garlic, ginger, and spices and sauté for about 1 minute.
3. Add 1 cup of the broth and bring to a boil.
4. Add the vegetables and again bring to a boil.
5. Cover the soup pan and cook for about 15–20 minutes, stirring occasionally.
6. Stir in the lemon juice and remove from the heat.
7. Serve hot with the topping of cashews and lemon zest.

Nutrition: Calories 425 Total Fat 32 g Saturated Fat 5.9 g Cholesterol 0 mg Sodium 601 mg Total Carbs 27.6 g Fiber 5.2 g Sugar 7.1 g Protein 13.4 g

300. Tofu with Brussels Sprouts

Preparation time: 15 minutes
Cooking time: 15 minutes
Servings: 3
Ingredients:

- 1½ tablespoons olive oil, divided
- 8 ounces' extra-firm tofu, drained, pressed, and cut into slices
- 2 garlic cloves, chopped
- 1/3 cup pecans, toasted, and chopped
- 1 tablespoon unsweetened applesauce
- ¼ cup fresh cilantro, chopped
- ½ pound Brussels sprouts, trimmed and cut into wide ribbons
- ¾ pound mixed bell peppers, seeded and sliced

Directions:
1. In a skillet, heat ½ tablespoon of the oil over medium heat and sauté the tofu and for about 6–7 minutes, or until golden-brown.
2. Add the garlic and pecans and sauté for about 1 minute.
3. Add the applesauce and cook for about 2 minutes.
4. Stir in the cilantro and remove from heat.
5. Transfer tofu into a plate and set aside
6. In the same skillet, heat the remaining oil over medium-high heat and cook the Brussels sprouts and bell peppers for about 5 minutes.
7. Stir in the tofu and remove from the heat.
8. Serve immediately.

Nutrition: Calories 238 Total Fat 17.8 g Saturated Fat 2 g Cholesterol 0 mg Sodium 26 mg Total Carbs 13.6 g Fiber 4.8 g Sugar 4.5 g Protein 11.8 g

301. Tofu with Peas

Preparation time: 15 minutes
Cooking time: 20 minutes

Servings: 5
Ingredients:

- 1 tablespoon chili-garlic sauce
- 3 tablespoons low-sodium soy sauce
- 2 tablespoons canola oil, divided
- 1 (16-ounce) package extra-firm tofu, drained, pressed, and cubed
- 1 cup yellow onion, chopped
- 1 tablespoon fresh ginger, minced
- 2 garlic cloves, minced
- 2 large tomatoes, chopped finely
- 5 cups frozen peas, thawed
- 1 teaspoon white sesame seeds

Directions:

1. For sauce: in a bowl, add the chili-garlic sauce and soy sauce and mix until well combined.
2. In a large skillet, heat 1 tablespoon of oil over medium-high heat and cook the tofu for about 4–5 minutes or until browned completely, stirring occasionally.
3. Transfer the tofu into a bowl.
4. In the same skillet, heat the remaining oil over medium heat and sauté the onion for about 3–4 minutes.
5. Add the ginger and garlic and sauté for about 1 minute.
6. Add the tomatoes and cook for about 4–5 minutes, crushing with the back of spoon.
7. Stir in all three peas and cook for about 2–3 minutes.
8. Stir in the sauce mixture and tofu and cook for about 1–2 minutes.
9. Serve hot with the garnishing of sesame seeds.

Nutrition: Calories 291 Total Fat 11.9 g Saturated Fat 1.1 g Cholesterol 0 mg Sodium 732 mg Total Carbs 31.6 g Fiber 10.8 g Sugar 11.5 g Protein 19 g

302. Carrot Soup with Tempeh

Preparation time: 15 minutes
Cooking time: 45 minutes
Servings: 6
Ingredients:

- ¼ cup olive oil, divided
- 1 large yellow onion, chopped
- Salt, to taste
- 2 pounds' carrots, peeled, and cut into ½-inch rounds
- 2 tablespoons fresh dill, chopped
- 4½ cups homemade vegetable broth
- 12 ounces' tempeh, cut into ½-inch cubes
- ¼ cup tomato paste
- 1 teaspoon fresh lemon juice

Directions:

1. In a large soup pan, heat 2 tablespoons of the oil over medium heat and cook the onion with salt for about 6–8 minutes, stirring frequently.
2. Add the carrots and stir to combine.
3. Lower the heat to low and cook, covered for about 5 minutes, stirring frequently.

4. Add in the broth and bring to a boil over high heat.
5. Lower the heat to a low and simmer, covered for about 30 minutes.
6. Meanwhile, in a skillet, heat the remaining oil over medium-high heat and cook the tempeh for about 3–5 minutes.
7. Stir in the dill and cook for about 1 minute.
8. Remove from the heat.
9. Remove the pan of soup from heat and stir in tomato paste and lemon juice.
10. With an immersion blender, blend the soup until smooth and creamy.
11. Serve the soup hot with the topping of tempeh.

Nutrition: Calories 294 Total Fat 15.7 g Saturated Fat 2.8 g Cholesterol 0 mg Sodium 723 mg Total Carbs 25.9 g Fiber 4.9 g Sugar 10.4 g Protein 16.4 g

303. Tempeh with Bell Peppers

Preparation time: 15 minutes
Cooking time: 15 minutes
Servings: 3
Ingredients:

- 2 tablespoons balsamic vinegar
- 2 tablespoons low-sodium soy sauce
- 2 tablespoons tomato sauce
- 1 teaspoon maple syrup
- ½ teaspoon garlic powder
- 1/8 teaspoon red pepper flakes, crushed
- 1 tablespoon vegetable oil
- 8 ounces' tempeh, cut into cubes
- 1 medium onion, chopped
- 2 large green bell peppers, seeded and chopped

Directions:

1. In a small bowl, add the vinegar, soy sauce, tomato sauce, maple syrup, garlic powder, and red pepper flakes and beat until well combined. Set aside.
2. Heat 1 tablespoon of oil in a large skillet over medium heat and cook the tempeh about 2–3 minutes per side.
3. Add the onion and bell peppers and heat for about 2–3 minutes.
4. Stir in the sauce mixture and cook for about 3–5 minutes, stirring frequently.
5. Serve hot.

Nutrition: Calories 241 Total Fat 13 g Saturated Fat 2.6 g Cholesterol 0 mg Sodium 65 mg Total Carbs 19.7 g Fiber 2.1 g Sugar 8.1 g Protein 16.1 g

304. Squash Medley

Preparation time: 10 minutes.
Cooking time: 20 minutes.
Servings: 2
Ingredients:

- 2lbs mixed squash
- 0.5 cup mixed veg
- 1 cup vegetable stock
- 2tbsp olive oil
- 2tbsp mixed herbs

Directions:

1. Put the squash in the steamer basket and add the stock into the Instant Pot.
2. Steam the squash in your Instant Pot for 10 minutes.
3. Depressurize and pour away the remaining stock.
4. Set to saute and add the oil and remaining ingredients.
5. Cook until a light crust forms.

Nutrition: Calories: 100 Carbs: 10 Sugar: 3 Fat: 6 Protein: 5 GL: 20

305. Eggplant Curry

Preparation time: 15 minutes
Cooking time: 20 minutes
Servings: 2
Ingredients:

- 2-3 cups chopped eggplant
- 1 thinly sliced onion
- 1 cup coconut milk
- 3tbsp curry paste
- 1tbsp oil or ghee

Directions:

1. Set the Instant Pot to saute and add the onion, oil, and curry paste.
2. When the onion is soft, add the remaining ingredients and seal.
3. Cook on Stew for 20 minutes.
4. Release the pressure naturally.

Nutrition: Calories: 350 Carbs: 15 Sugar: 3 Fat: 25 Protein: 11 GL: 10

306. Chickpea Soup

Preparation time: 15 minutes
Cooking time: 35 minutes
Servings: 2
Ingredients:

- 1lb cooked chickpeas
- 1lb chopped vegetables
- 1 cup low sodium vegetable broth
- 2tbsp mixed herbs

Directions:

1. Mix all the ingredients in your Instant Pot.
2. Cook on Stew for 35 minutes.
3. Release the pressure naturally.

Nutrition: Calories: 310 Carbs: 20 Sugar: 3 Fat: 5 Protein: 27 GL: 5

307. Fried Tofu Hotpot

Preparation time: 15 minutes
Cooking time: 15 minutes
Servings: 2
Ingredients:

- 0.5lb fried tofu
- 1lb chopped Chinese vegetable mix
- 1 cup low sodium vegetable broth
- 2tbsp 5 spice seasoning
- 1tbsp smoked paprika

Directions:

1. Mix all the ingredients in your Instant Pot.
2. Cook on Stew for 15 minutes.
3. Release the pressure naturally.

Nutrition: Calories: 320 Carbs: 11 Sugar: 3 Fat: 23 Protein: 47 GL: 6

308. Pea and Mint Soup

Preparation time: 15 minutes
Cooking time: 35 minutes
Servings: 2
Ingredients:

- 1lb green peas
- 2 cups low sodium vegetable broth
- 3tbsp mint sauce

Directions:

1. Mix all the ingredients in your Instant Pot.
2. Cook on Stew for 35 minutes.
3. Release the pressure naturally.
4. Blend into a rough soup.

Nutrition: Calories: 130 Carbs: 17 Sugar: 4 Fat: 5 Protein: 19 GL: 11

309. Lentil and Eggplant Stew

Preparation time: 15 minutes
Cooking time: 35 minutes
Servings: 2
Ingredients:

- 1lb eggplant
- 1lb dry lentils
- 1 cup chopped vegetables
- 1 cup low sodium vegetable broth

Directions:

1. Mix all the ingredients in your Instant Pot.
2. Cook on Stew for 35 minutes.
3. Release the pressure naturally.

Nutrition: Calories: 310 Carbs: 22 Sugar: 6 Fat: 10 Protein: 32 GL: 16

310. Tofu Curry

Preparation time: 15 minutes
Cooking time: 20 minutes
Servings: 2
Ingredients:

- 2 cups cubed extra firm tofu
- 2 cups mixed stir fry vegetables
- 0.5 cup soy yogurt
- 3tbsp curry paste
- 1tbsp oil or ghee

Directions:

1. Set the Instant Pot to saute and add the oil and curry paste.
2. When the onion is soft, add the remaining ingredients except the yogurt and seal.
3. Cook on Stew for 20 minutes.
4. Release the pressure naturally and serve with a scoop of soy yogurt.

Nutrition: Calories: 300 Carbs: 9 Sugar: 4 Fat: 14 Protein: 42 GL: 7

311. Fake On-Stew

Preparation time: 15 minutes
Cooking time: 25 minutes
Servings: 2
Ingredients:

- 0.5lb soy bacon
- 1lb chopped vegetables
- 1 cup low sodium vegetable broth
- 1tbsp nutritional yeast

Directions:
1. Mix all the ingredients in your Instant Pot.
2. Cook on Stew for 25 minutes.
3. Release the pressure naturally.

Nutrition: Calories: 200 Carbs: 12 Sugar: 3 Fat: 7 Protein: 41 GL: 5

312. Lentil and Chickpea Curry

Preparation time: 15 minutes
Cooking time: 20 minutes
Servings: 2
Ingredients:

- 2 cups dry lentils and chickpeas
- 1 thinly sliced onion
- 1 cup chopped tomato
- 3tbsp curry paste
- 1tbsp oil or ghee

Directions:
1. Set the Instant Pot to saute and add the onion, oil, and curry paste.
2. When the onion is soft, add the remaining ingredients and seal.
3. Cook on Stew for 20 minutes.
4. Release the pressure naturally.

Nutrition: Calories: 360 Carbs: 26 Sugar: 6 Fat: 19 Protein: 23 GL: 10

313. Seitan Roast

Preparation time: 15 minutes
Cooking time: 35 minutes
Servings: 2
Ingredients:

- 1lb seitan roulade
- 1lb chopped winter vegetables
- 1 cup low sodium vegetable broth
- 4tbsp roast rub

Directions:
1. Rub the roast rub into your roulade.
2. Place the roulade and vegetables in your Instant Pot.
3. Add the broth. Seal.
4. Cook on Stew for 35 minutes.
5. Release the pressure naturally.

Nutrition: Calories: 260 Carbs: 9 Sugar: 2 Fat: 2 Protein: 49 GL: 4

314. Zucchini with Tomatoes

Preparation Time: 15 minutes
Cooking Time: 11 minutes
Servings: 8
Ingredients:

- 6 medium zucchinis, chopped roughly
- 1-pound cherry tomatoes
- 2 small onions, chopped roughly
- 2 tablespoons fresh basil, chopped
- 1 cup water

- 1 tablespoon olive oil
- 2 garlic cloves, minced
- Salt and ground black pepper, as required

Directions:
1. In the Instant Pot, place oil and press "Sauté". Now add the onion, garlic, ginger, and spices and cook for about 3-4 minutes.
2. Add the zucchinis and tomatoes and cook for about 1-2 minutes.
3. Press "Cancel" and stir in the remaining ingredients except basil.
4. Close the lid and place the pressure valve to "Seal" position.
5. Press "Manual" and cook under "High Pressure" for about 5 minutes.
6. Press "Cancel" and allow a "Natural" release.
7. Open the lid and transfer the vegetable mixture onto a serving platter.
8. Garnish with basil and serve.

Nutrition: Calories: 57 Fats: 2.1g Carbohydrates: 9gSugar: 4.8gProteins: 2.5g Sodium: 39mg

315. Asian Fried Eggplant

Preparation Time: 10 minutes
Cooking Time: 40 minutes
Servings: 4
Ingredients:

- 1 large eggplant, sliced into fourths
- 3 green onions, diced, green tips only
- 1 teaspoon fresh ginger, peeled & diced fine
- ¼ cup + 1 teaspoon cornstarch
- 1 ½ tablespoon. soy sauce
- 1 ½ tablespoon. sesame oil
- 1 tablespoon. vegetable oil
- 1 tablespoon. fish sauce
- 2 teaspoon Splenda
- ¼ teaspoon salt

Directions:
1. Place eggplant on paper towels and sprinkle both sides with salt. Let for 1 hour to remove excess moisture. Pat dry with more paper towels.
2. In a small bowl, whisk together soy sauce, sesame oil, fish sauce, Splenda, and 1 teaspoon cornstarch.
3. Coat both sides of the eggplant with the ¼ cup cornstarch, use more if needed.
4. Heat oil in a large skillet, over med-high heat. Add ½ the ginger and 1 green onion, then lay 2 slices of eggplant on top. Use ½ the sauce mixture to lightly coat both sides of the eggplant. Cook 8-10 minutes per side. Repeat.
5. Serve garnished with remaining green onions.

Nutrition: Calories 155 Total Carbohydrates 18g Net Carbohydrates 13g Protein 2g Fat 9g Sugar 6g Fiber 5g

316. Butternut fritters

Preparation Time: 15 minutes
Cooking Time: 15 minutes
Servings: 6
Ingredients:

- 5 cup butternut squash, grated

- 2 large eggs
- 1 tablespoon. fresh sage, diced fine
- 2/3 cup flour
- 2 tablespoons olive oil
- Salt and pepper, to taste

Directions:

1. Heat oil in a large skillet over med-high heat.
2. In a large bowl, combine squash, eggs, sage and salt and pepper to taste. Fold in flour.
3. Drop ¼ cup mixture into skillet, keeping fritters at least 1 inch apart. Cook till golden brown on both sides, about 2 minutes per side.
4. Transfer to paper towel lined plate. Repeat. Serve immediately with your favorite dipping sauce.

Nutrition: Calories 164 Total Carbohydrates 24g Net Carbohydrates 21g Protein 4g Fat 6g Sugar 3g Fiber 3g

317. Cauliflower Mushroom Risotto

Preparation Time: 10 minutes
Cooking Time: 30 minutes
Servings: 2
Ingredients:

- 1 medium head cauliflower, grated
- 8-ounce Porcini mushrooms, sliced
- 1 yellow onion, diced fine
- 2 cup low sodium vegetable broth
- 2 teaspoon garlic, diced fine
- 2 teaspoon white wine vinegar
- Salt & pepper, to taste
- Olive oil cooking spray

Directions:

1. Heat oven to 350 degrees. Line a baking sheet with foil.
2. Place the mushrooms on the prepared pan and spray with cooking spray. Sprinkle with salt and toss to coat. Bake 10-12 minutes, or until golden brown and the mushrooms start to crisp.
3. Spray a large skillet with cooking spray and place over med-high heat. Add onion and cook, stirring frequently, until translucent, about 3-4 minutes. Add garlic and cook 2 minutes, until golden.
4. Add the cauliflower and cook 1 minute, stirring.
5. Place the broth in a saucepan and bring to a simmer. Add to the skillet, ¼ cup at a time, mixing well after each addition.
6. Stir in vinegar. Reduce heat to low and let simmer, 4-5 minutes, or until most of the liquid has evaporated.
7. Spoon cauliflower mixture onto plates, or in bowls, and top with mushrooms. Serve.

Nutrition: Calories 134 Total Carbohydrates 22g Protein 10g Fat 0g Sugar 5g Fiber 2g

318. Chili Sin Carne

Preparation time: 15 minutes
Cooking time: 35 minutes
Servings: 2
Ingredients:

- 3 cups mixed cooked beans

- 2 cups chopped tomatoes
- 1tbsp yeast extract
- 2 squares very dark chocolate
- 1tbsp red chili flakes

Directions:

1. Mix all the ingredients in your Instant Pot.
2. Cook on Beans for 35 minutes.
3. Release the pressure naturally.

Nutrition: Calories: 240 Carbs: 20 Sugar: 5 Fat: 3 Protein: 36 GL: 11

319. Meatless Ball Soup

Preparation time: 15 minutes
Cooking time: 15 minutes
Servings: 2
Ingredients:

- 1lb minced tofu
- 0.5lb chopped vegetables
- 2 cups low sodium vegetable broth
- 1tbsp almond flour
- salt and pepper

Directions:

1. Mix the tofu, flour, salt and pepper.
2. Form the meatballs.
3. Place all the ingredients in your Instant Pot.
4. Cook on Stew for 15 minutes.
5. Release the pressure naturally.

Nutrition: Calories: 240 Carbs: 9 Sugar: 3 Fat: 10 Protein: 35 GL: 5

320. Seitan Curry

Preparation time: 15 minutes
Cooking time: 20 minutes
Servings: 2
Ingredients:

- 0.5lb seitan
- 1 thinly sliced onion
- 1 cup chopped tomato
- 3tbsp curry paste
- 1tbsp oil or ghee

Directions:

1. Set the Instant Pot to saute and add the onion, oil, and curry paste.
2. When the onion is soft, add the remaining ingredients and seal.
3. Cook on Stew for 20 minutes.
4. Release the pressure naturally.

Nutrition: Calories: 240 Carbs: 19 Sugar: 4 Fat: 10 Protein: 32 GL: 10

321. Split Pea Stew

Preparation time: 5 minutes
Cooking time: 35 minutes
Servings: 2
Ingredients:

- 1 cup dry split peas
- 1lb chopped vegetables
- 1 cup mushroom soup
- 2tbsp old bay seasoning

Directions:

1. Mix all the ingredients in your Instant Pot.
2. Cook on Beans for 35 minutes.
3. Release the pressure naturally.

Nutrition: Calories: 300 Carbs: 7 Sugar: 3 Fat: 2 Protein: 24 GL: 4

322. <u>Mango Tofu Curry</u>

Preparation time: 15 minutes
Cooking time: 35 minutes
Servings: 2
Ingredients:

- 1lb cubed extra firm tofu
- 1lb chopped vegetables
- 1 cup low carb mango sauce
- 1 cup vegetable broth
- 2tbsp curry paste

Directions:

1. Mix all the ingredients in your Instant Pot.
2. Cook on Stew for 35 minutes.
3. Release the pressure naturally.

Nutrition: Calories: 310 Carbs: 20 Sugar: 9 Fat: 4 Protein: 37 GL: 19

323. <u>Cauliflower in Vegan Alfredo Sauce</u>

Preparation time: 15 minutes
Cooking time: 35 minutes
Servings: 1
Ingredients:

- Olive oil: 1 tablespoon
- Garlic: 2 cloves
- Vegetable broth: 1 cup
- Sea salt: ½ teaspoon
- Pepper: as per taste
- Chilli flakes: 1 teaspoon
- Onion (diced): 1 medium
- Cauliflower florets (chopped): 4 cups
- Lemon juice (freshly squeezed): 1 teaspoon
- Nutritional yeast: 1 tablespoon
- Vegan butter: 2 tablespoons
- Zucchini noodles: for serving

Directions:

1. Begin by positioning a cooking pot on low heat. Stream in the oil and allow it to heat through.
2. Immediately you're done, toss in the chopped onion and set on fire for about 4 minutes. The onion should be translucent.
3. Put in the garlic and Prepare for about 30 seconds. Continuously stir to prevent them from sticking.
4. Put in the vegetable broth and shredded cauliflower florets. Ensure you mix well and cover the stockpot with a lid. Allow the cauliflower cook for 5 minutes and then extract it from the flame.
5. Get a blender and move the cooked cauliflower into it. Palpitate until the puree is smooth and creamy in texture. (Add 1 tablespoon of broth if required for.)
6. Put salt, lemon juice, nutritional yeast, butter, chilli flakes, and pepper to the blender. Mix until all the ingredients fully combine to form a smooth puree.
7. Position the zucchini noodles over a dishing platter and stream the Prepare cauliflower Alfredo sauce over the noodles.

Nutrition: Fat: 9.1 g Protein: 3.9 g Carbohydrates: 10 g

324. <u>Tomato and Zucchini Sauté</u>

Preparation time: 15 minutes
Cooking time: 35 minutes
Servings: 6
Ingredients:

- Vegetable oil: 1 tablespoon
- Tomatoes (chopped): 2
- Green bell pepper (chopped): 1
- Black pepper (freshly ground): as per taste
- Onion (sliced): 1
- Zucchini (peeled): 2 pounds and cut into 1-inch-thick slices
- Salt: as per taste
- Uncooked white rice: ¼ cup

Directions:

1. Begin by getting a nonstick pan and putting it over low heat. Stream in the oil and allow it to heat through.
2. Put in the onions and sauté for about 3 minutes.
3. Then pour in the zucchini and green peppers. Mix well and spice with black pepper and salt.
4. Reduce the heat and cover the pan with a lid. Allow the veggies cook on low for 5 minutes.
5. While you're done, put in the water and rice. Place the lid back on and cook on low for 20 minutes.

Nutrition: Fat: 2.8 g Protein: 3.2 g Carbohydrates: 16.1 g

325. <u>Steamed Kale with Mediterranean Dressing</u>

Preparation time: 15 minutes
Cooking time: 35 minutes
Servings: 6
Ingredients:

- Kale (chopped): 12 cups
- Olive oil: 1 tablespoon
- Soy sauce: 1 teaspoon
- Pepper (freshly ground): as per taste
- Lemon juice: 2 tablespoons
- Garlic (minced): 1 tablespoon
- Salt: as per taste

Directions:

1. Get a gas steamer or an electric steamer and fill the bottom pan with water. If making use of a gas steamer, position it on high heat. Making use of an electric steamer, place it on the highest setting.
2. Immediately the water comes to a boil, put in the shredded kale and cover with a lid. Boil for about 8 minutes. The kale should be tender by now.
3. During the kale is boiling, take a big mixing bowl and put in the olive oil, lemon juice, soy sauce, garlic, pepper, and salt. Whisk well to mix.
4. Now toss in the steamed kale and carefully enclose into the dressing. Be assured the kale is well-coated.
5. Serve while it's hot!

Nutrition: Fat: 3.5 g Protein: 4.6 g Carbohydrates: 14.5 g

326. <u>Healthy Carrot Muffins</u>

Preparation time: 15 minutes
Cooking time: 30 minutes
Servings: 1
Ingredients:

- Tapioca starch: ¼ cup
- Baking soda: 1 teaspoon
- Cinnamon: 1 tablespoon
- Cloves: ¼ teaspoon
- Wet ingredients
- Vanilla extract: 1 teaspoon
- Water: 1½ cups
- Carrots (shredded): 1½ cups
- Almond flour: 1¾ cups
- Granulated sweetener of choice: ½ cup
- Baking powder: 1 teaspoon
- Nutmeg: 1 teaspoon
- Salt: 1 teaspoon
- Coconut oil: 1/3 cup
- Flax meal: 4 tablespoons
- Banana (mashed): 1 medium

Directions:

1. Begin by heating the oven to 350°F.
2. Get a muffin tray and position paper cups in all the moulds. Arrange aside.
3. Get a small glass bowl and put half a cup of water and flax meal. Allow this rest for about 5 minutes.
4. Get a large mixing bowl and put in the almond flour, tapioca starch, granulated sugar, baking soda, baking powder, cinnamon, nutmeg, cloves, and salt. Mix well to combine.
5. Conform a well in the middle of the flour mixture and stream in the coconut oil, vanilla extract, and flax egg. Mix well to conform a mushy dough.
6. Then put in the chopped carrots and mashed banana. Mix until well-combined.
7. Make use of a spoon to scoop out an equal amount of mixture into 8 muffin cups.
8. Position the muffin tray in the oven and allow it to bake for about 40 minutes.
9. Extract the tray from the microwave and allow the muffins to stand for about 10 minutes.
10. Extract the muffin cups from the tray and allow them to chill until they reach room degree of hotness and coldness.
11. Serve and enjoy!

Nutrition: Fat: 13.9 g Protein: 3.8 g Carbohydrates: 17.3 g

327. <u>Vegetable Noodles Stir-Fry</u>

Preparation time: 5 minutes
Cooking time: 35 minutes
Servings: 1
Ingredients:

- White sweet potato: 1 pound
- Zucchini: 8 ounces
- Garlic cloves (finely chopped): 2 large
- Vegetable broth: 2 tablespoons

- Salt: as per taste
- Carrots: 8 ounces
- Shallot (finely chopped): 1
- Red chilli (finely chopped): 1
- Olive oil: 1 tablespoon
- Pepper: as per taste

Directions:

1. Begin by scrapping the carrots and sweet potato. Make Use a spiralizer to make noodles out of the sweet potato and carrots.
2. Rinse the zucchini thoroughly and spiralize it as well.
3. Get a large skillet and position it on a high flame. Stream in the vegetable broth and allow it to come to a boil.
4. Toss in the spiralized sweet potato and carrots. Then put in the chilli, garlic, and shallots. Stir everything using tongs and cook for some minutes.
5. Transfer the vegetable noodles into a serving platter and generously spice with pepper and salt.
6. Finalize by sprinkling olive oil over the noodles. Serve while hot!

Nutrition: Fat: 3.7 g Protein: 3.6 g Carbohydrates: 31.2 g

328. <u>Black Bean and Veggie Soup Topped with Lime Salsa</u>

Preparation time: 15 minutes
Cooking time: 35 minutes
Servings: 1
Ingredients:

- Onions (diced): 2
- Celery (diced): 3 sticks
- Garlic (finely chopped): 3 cloves
- Cilantro: ½ bunch
- Dried oregano: 1 tablespoon
- Sea salt: ½ tablespoon
- Boiling water: 1 quart
- Salad onion (finely chopped): ½ small
- Carrots (diced): 2
- Red bell peppers (diced): 2
- Red chilis (remove seed): 2
- Bay leaf: 1
- Black pepper (freshly ground): 1 tablespoon
- Black beans (drained and rinsed): 2 cans (15 ounces)
- Tomato (finely chopped): 1
- Fresh juice of ½ lime

Directions:

1. Begin by extracting the leaves and stalks from the cilantro. Neatly shred the stalks and leaves. Arrange aside
2. Ge a large saucepan and stream in 3 tablespoons of water. In this, put the carrots, onions, bell peppers, celery, red chillies, garlic, coriander stalks, oregano, bay leaf, sea salt, and pepper. Mix until well-combined. Cover the pan using a lid and allow the veggies to cook for about 10 minutes. Keep mixing.
3. Put the black beans and boiling water into the saucepan. Keep stirring.

4. Extract the lid from the saucepan and low heat. Allow the soup to cook for half a minute.
5. While the soup is on a high flame, form the lime salsa. In this, you will mix the tomato, salad onion, and cilantro leaves in a small bowl. Crush in the fresh lime juice.
6. Stream the soup in a big and deep bowl and finish by topping with lime salsa.

Nutrition: Fat: 2.4 g Protein: 17.2 g Carbohydrates: 53.9 g

329. **Cauliflower and Kabocha Squash Soup**

Preparation time: 15 minutes
Cooking time: 35 minutes
Servings: 1
Ingredients:

- Olive oil: 2 tablespoons
- Garlic (minced): 3 cloves
- Cauliflower florets: 2½ cups
- Ground cardamom: ½ teaspoon
- Bay leaves: 2
- Vanilla almond milk (unsweetened): ½ cup
- Pepper: ¼ teaspoon
- Yellow onion (diced): ½
- Fresh ginger (minced): 1 tablespoon
- Kabocha squash (cubed): 2½ cups
- Cayenne: ¼ teaspoon
- Vegetable broth: 4 cups
- Salt: ½ teaspoon

Directions:

1. Begin by streaming the olive oil into a nonstick saucepan and position it over a high flame.
2. Toss in the onion, ginger, and garlic. Sauté for around 3 minutes.
3. Then put in the squash, cauliflower, cayenne, bay leaves, and cardamom. Combine well.
4. Stream in the vegetable broth and take the vegetables and stock mixture to a boil.
5. Reduce the flame and allow the soup simmer for 10 minutes.
6. Extract the pan and use the blender to puree the mixture.
7. Immediately the soup is pureed, replace the pan to the low heat. Put in the almond milk. Combine well.
8. Finalize by spicing with pepper and salt.

Nutrition: Fat: 7.7 g Protein: 3.4 g Carbohydrates: 11.6 g

330. **Easy Brussels Sprouts Hash**

Preparation Time: 20 minutes
Cooking Time: 10 minutes
Servings: 4
Ingredients:

- 3 tablespoons extra-virgin olive oil
- 1 onion, finely chopped
- 1 pound Brussels sprouts, bottoms trimmed off, shredded (see tip)
- ½ teaspoon caraway seeds
- ½ teaspoon sea salt
- ⅛ teaspoon freshly ground black pepper

- ¼ cup red wine vinegar
- 1 tablespoon Dijon mustard
- 1 tablespoon honey
- 3 garlic cloves, minced

Directions:

1. In a large skillet over medium-high heat, heat the olive oil until it shimmers.
2. Add the onion, Brussels sprouts, caraway seeds, sea salt, and pepper. Cook for 7 to 10 minutes, stirring occasionally, until the Brussels sprouts begin to brown.
3. While the Brussels sprouts cook, whisk the vinegar, mustard, and honey in a small bowl and set aside.
4. Add the garlic to the skillet and cook for 30 seconds, stirring constantly.
5. Add the vinegar mixture to the skillet. Cook for about 5 minutes, stirring, until the liquid reduces by half.

Nutrition: Calories: 176; Protein: 11g; Total Carbohydrates: 19g; Sugars: 8g; Fiber: 5g; Total Fat: 11g; Saturated Fat: 1g; Cholesterol: 0mg; Sodium: 309mg

331. **Roasted Asparagus with Lemon and Pine Nuts**

Preparation Time: 5 minutes
Cooking Time: 20 minutes
Servings: 4
Ingredients:

- 1-pound asparagus, trimmed
- 2 tablespoons extra-virgin olive oil
- Juice of 1 lemon
- Zest of 1 lemon
- ¼ cup pine nuts
- ½ teaspoon sea salt
- ⅛ teaspoon freshly ground black pepper

Directions:

1. Preheat the oven to 425°F.
2. In a large bowl, toss the asparagus with the olive oil, lemon juice and zest, pine nuts, sea salt, and pepper. Spread in a roasting pan in an even layer.
3. Roast for about 20 minutes until the asparagus is browned.

Nutrition: Calories: 144; Protein: 4g; Total Carbohydrates: 6g; Sugars: 3g; Fiber: 3g; Total Fat: 13g;Saturated Fat: 1g; Cholesterol: 0mg; Sodium: 240mg

332. **Citrus Sautéed Spinach**

Preparation Time: 5 minutes
Cooking Time: 5 minutes
Servings: 4
Ingredients:

- 2 tablespoons extra-virgin olive oil
- 4 cups fresh baby spinach
- 1 teaspoon orange zest
- ¼ cup freshly squeezed orange juice
- ½ teaspoon sea salt
- ⅛ teaspoon freshly ground black pepper

Directions:

1. In a large skillet over medium-high heat, heat the olive oil until it shimmers.
2. Add the spinach and orange zest. Cook for about 3 minutes, stirring occasionally, until the spinach wilts.
3. Stir in the orange juice, sea salt, and pepper. Cook for 2 minutes more, stirring occasionally. Serve hot.

Nutrition: Calories: 74; Protein: 7g; Total Carbohydrates: 3g; Sugars: 1g; Fiber: 1g; Total Fat: 7g; Saturated Fat: 1g;Cholesterol: 0mg;Sodium: 258mg

333. **Mashed Cauliflower**

Preparation Time: 10 minutes
Cooking Time: 15 minutes
Servings: 4
Ingredients:

- 4 cups cauliflower florets
- ¼ cup skim milk
- ¼ cup (2 ounces) grated Parmesan cheese
- 2 tablespoons butter
- 2 tablespoons extra-virgin olive oil
- ½ teaspoon sea salt
- ⅛ teaspoon freshly ground black pepper

Directions:

1. In a large pot over medium-high, cover the cauliflower with water and bring it to a boil. Reduce the heat to medium-low, cover, and simmer for about 10 minutes until the cauliflower is soft.
2. Drain the cauliflower and return it to the pot. Add the milk, cheese, butter, olive oil, sea salt, and pepper. Using a potato masher, mash until smooth.

Nutrition: Calories: 187; Protein: 7g; Total Carbohydrates: 7g; Sugars: 3g; Fiber: 3g; Total Fat: 16g; Saturated Fat: 7g; Cholesterol: 26mg; Sodium: 445mg

334. **Broccoli with Ginger and Garlic**

Preparation Time: 10 minutes
Cooking Time: 11 minutes
Servings: 4
Ingredients:

- 2 tablespoons extra-virgin olive oil
- 2 cups broccoli florets
- 1 tablespoon grated fresh ginger
- ½ teaspoon sea salt
- ⅛ teaspoon freshly ground black pepper
- 3 garlic cloves, minced

Directions:

1. In a large skillet over medium-high heat, heat the olive oil until it shimmers.
2. Add the broccoli, ginger, sea salt, and pepper. Cook for about 10 minutes, stirring occasionally, until the broccoli is soft and starts to brown.
3. Add the garlic and cook for 30 seconds, stirring constantly. Remove from the heat and serve.

Nutrition: Per Serving Calories: 80; Protein: 1g; Total Carbohydrates: 4g; Sugars: 1g; Fiber: 1g; Total Fat: 0g; Saturated Fat: 1g; Cholesterol: 0mg; Sodium: 249mg

335. **Balsamic Roasted Carrots**

Preparation Time: 10 minutes
Cooking Time: 30 minutes
Servings: 4
Ingredients:

- 1½ pounds carrots, quartered lengthwise
- 2 tablespoons extra-virgin olive oil
- ¼ teaspoon sea salt
- ⅛ teaspoon freshly ground black pepper
- 3 tablespoons balsamic vinegar

Directions:

1. Preheat the oven to 425°F.
2. In a large bowl, toss the carrots with the olive oil, sea salt, and pepper. Place in a single layer in a roasting pan or on a rimmed baking sheet. Roast for 20 to 30 minutes until the carrots are caramelized.
3. Toss with the vinegar and serve.

Nutrition: Calories: 132; Protein: 1g; Total Carbohydrates: 17g; Sugars: 8g; Fiber: 4g; Total Fat: 7g; Saturated Fat: 1g; Cholesterol: 0mg; Sodium: 235mg

SOUP AND STEW RECIPES

336. Delicious Chicken Soup

Preparation Time: 10 minutes
Cooking Time: 4 hours 30 minutes
Servings: 4
Ingredients:

- 1 lb chicken breasts, boneless and skinless
- 2 Tbsp fresh basil, chopped
- 1 1/2 cups mozzarella cheese, shredded
- 2 garlic cloves, minced
- 1 Tbsp Parmesan cheese, grated
- 2 Tbsp dried basil
- 2 cups chicken stock
- 28 oz tomatoes, diced
- 1/4 tsp pepper
- 1/2 tsp salt

Directions:

1. Add chicken, Parmesan cheese, dried basil, tomatoes, garlic, pepper, and salt to a crock pot and stir well to combine.
2. Cover and cook on low for 4 hours.
3. Add fresh basil and mozzarella cheese and stir well.
4. Cover again and cook for 30 more minutes or until cheese is melted.
5. Remove chicken from the crock pot and shred using forks.
6. Return shredded chicken to the crock pot and stir to mix.
7. Serve and enjoy.

Nutrition: Calories 299 Fat 11.6 g Carbohydrates 9.3 g Sugar 5.6 g Protein 38.8 g Cholesterol 108 mg

337. Flavorful Broccoli Soup

Preparation Time: 10 minutes
Cooking Time: 4 hours 15 minutes
Servings: 6
Ingredients:

- 20 oz broccoli florets
- 4 oz cream cheese
- 8 oz cheddar cheese, shredded
- 1/2 tsp paprika
- 1/2 tsp ground mustard
- 3 cups chicken stock
- 2 garlic cloves, chopped
- 1 onion, diced
- 1 cup carrots, shredded
- 1/4 tsp baking soda
- 1/4 tsp salt

Directions:

1. Add all ingredients except cream cheese and cheddar cheese to a crock pot and stir well.
2. Cover and cook on low for 4 hours.
3. Purée the soup using an immersion blender until smooth.
4. Stir in the cream cheese and cheddar cheese.
5. Cover and cook on low for 15 minutes longer.

6. Season with pepper and salt.
7. Serve and enjoy.

Nutrition: Calories 275 Fat 19.9 g Carbohydrates 11.9 g Sugar 4 g Protein 14.4 g Cholesterol 60 mg

338. Healthy Chicken Kale Soup

Preparation Time: 10 minutes
Cooking Time: 6 hours 15 minutes
Servings: 6
Ingredients:

- 2 lb chicken breasts, skinless and boneless
- 1/4 cup fresh lemon juice
- 5 oz baby kale
- 32 oz chicken stock
- 1/2 cup olive oil
- 1 large onion, sliced
- 14 oz chicken broth
- 1 Tbsp extra-virgin olive oil
- Salt

Directions:

1. Heat the extra-virgin olive oil in a pan over medium heat.
2. Season chicken with salt and place in the hot pan.
3. Cover pan and cook chicken for 15 minutes.
4. Remove chicken from the pan and shred it using forks.
5. Add shredded chicken to a crock pot.
6. Add sliced onion, olive oil, and broth to a blender and blend until combined.
7. Pour blended mixture into the crock pot.
8. Add remaining ingredients to the crock pot and stir well.
9. Cover and cook on low for 6 hours.
10. Stir well and serve.

Nutrition: Calories 493 Fat 31.3 g Carbohydrates 5.8 g Sugar 1.9 g Protein 46.7 g Cholesterol 135 mg

339. Spicy Chicken Pepper Stew

Preparation Time: 10 minutes
Cooking Time: 6 hours
Servings: 6
Ingredients:

- 3 chicken breasts, skinless and boneless, cut into small pieces
- 1 tsp garlic, minced
- 1 tsp ground ginger
- 2 tsp olive oil
- 2 tsp soy sauce
- 1 Tbsp fresh lemon juice
- 1/2 cup green onions, sliced
- 1 Tbsp crushed red pepper
- 8 oz chicken stock
- 1 bell pepper, chopped
- 1 green chili pepper, sliced
- 2 jalapeño peppers, sliced
- 1/2 tsp black pepper

- 1/4 tsp sea salt

Directions:
1. Add all ingredients to a large mixing bowl and mix well. Place in the refrigerator overnight.
2. Pour marinated chicken mixture into a crock pot.
3. Cover and cook on low for 6 hours.
4. Stir well and serve.

Nutrition: Calories 171 Fat 7.4 g Carbohydrates 3.7 g Sugar 1.7 g Protein 22 g Cholesterol 65 mg

340. Beef Chili

Preparation Time: 10 minutes
Cooking Time: 8 hours
Servings: 6
Ingredients:
- 1 lb ground beef
- 1 tsp garlic powder
- 1 tsp paprika
- 3 tsp chili powder
- 1 Tbsp Worcestershire sauce
- 1 Tbsp fresh parsley, chopped
- 1 tsp onion powder
- 25 oz tomatoes, chopped
- 4 carrots, chopped
- 1 onion, diced
- 1 bell pepper, diced
- 1/2 tsp sea salt

Directions:
1. Brown the ground meat in a pan over high heat until meat is no longer pink.
2. Transfer meat to a crock pot.
3. Add bell pepper, tomatoes, carrots, and onion to the crock pot and stir well.
4. Add remaining ingredients and stir well.
5. Cover and cook on low for 8 hours.
6. Serve and enjoy.

Nutrition: Calories 152 Fat 4 g Carbohydrates 10.4 g Sugar 5.8 g Protein 18.8 g Cholesterol 51 mg

341. Tasty Basil Tomato Soup

Preparation Time: 10 minutes
Cooking Time: 6 hours
Servings: 6
Ingredients:
- 28 oz can whole peeled tomatoes
- 1/2 cup fresh basil leaves
- 4 cups chicken stock
- 1 tsp red pepper flakes
- 3 garlic cloves, peeled
- 2 onions, diced
- 3 carrots, peeled and diced
- 3 Tbsp olive oil
- 1 tsp salt

Directions:
1. Add all ingredients to a crock pot and stir well.
2. Cover and cook on low for 6 hours.
3. Purée the soup until smooth using an immersion blender.
4. Season soup with pepper and salt.

5. Serve and enjoy.

Nutrition: Calories 126 Fat 7.5 g Carbohydrates 13.3 g Sugar 7 g Protein 2.5 g Cholesterol 0 mg

342. Healthy Spinach Soup

Preparation Time: 10 minutes
Cooking Time: 3 hours
Servings: 8
Ingredients:
- 3 cups frozen spinach, chopped, thawed and drained
- 8 oz cheddar cheese, shredded
- 1 egg, lightly beaten
- 10 oz can cream of chicken soup
- 8 oz cream cheese, softened

Directions:
1. Add spinach to a large bowl. Purée the spinach.
2. Add egg, chicken soup, cream cheese, and pepper to the spinach purée and mix well.
3. Transfer spinach mixture to a crock pot.
4. Cover and cook on low for 3 hours.
5. Stir in cheddar cheese and serve.

Nutrition: Calories 256 Fat 21.9 g Carbohydrates 4.1 g Sugar 0.5 g Protein 11.1 g Cholesterol 84 mg

343. Mexican Chicken Soup

Preparation Time: 10 minutes
Cooking Time: 4 hours
Servings: 6
Ingredients:
- 1 1/2 lb chicken thighs, skinless and boneless
- 14 oz chicken stock
- 14 oz salsa
- 8 oz Monterey Jack cheese, shredded

Directions:
1. Place chicken into a crock pot.
2. Pour remaining ingredients over the chicken.
3. Cover and cook on high for 4 hours.
4. Remove chicken from crock pot and shred using forks.
5. Return shredded chicken to the crock pot and stir well.
6. Serve and enjoy.

Nutrition: Calories 371 Fat 19.5 g Carbohydrates 5.7 g Sugar 2.2 g Protein 42.1 g Cholesterol 135 mg

344. Beef Stew

Preparation Time: 10 minutes
Cooking Time: 5 hours 5 minutes
Servings: 8
Ingredients:
- 3 lb beef stew meat, trimmed
- 1/2 cup red curry paste
- 1/3 cup tomato paste
- 13 oz can coconut milk
- 2 tsp ginger, minced
- 2 garlic cloves, minced
- 1 medium onion, sliced
- 2 Tbsp olive oil
- 2 cups carrots, julienned

- 2 cups broccoli florets
- 2 tsp fresh lime juice
- 2 Tbsp fish sauce
- 2 tsp sea salt

Directions:
1. Heat 1 tablespoon of oil in a pan over medium heat.
2. Brown the meat on all sides in the pan.
3. Add brown meat to a crock pot.
4. Add remaining oil to the same pan and sauté the ginger, garlic, and onion over medium-high heat for 5 minutes.
5. Add coconut milk and stir well.
6. Transfer pan mixture to the crock pot.
7. Add remaining ingredients except for carrots and broccoli.
8. Cover and cook on high for 5 hours.
9. Add carrots and broccoli during the last 30 minutes of cooking.
10. Serve and enjoy.

Nutrition: Calories 537 Fat 28.6 g Carbohydrates 13 g Sugar 12.6 g Protein 54.4 g Cholesterol 152 mg

345. Creamy Broccoli Cauliflower Soup

Preparation Time: 10 minutes
Cooking Time: 6 hours
Servings: 6
Ingredients:

- 2 cups cauliflower florets, chopped
- 3 cups broccoli florets, chopped
- 3 1/2 cups chicken stock
- 1 large carrot, diced
- 1/2 cup shallots, diced
- 2 garlic cloves, minced
- 1 cup plain yogurt
- 6 oz cheddar cheese, shredded
- 1 cup coconut milk
- Pepper
- Salt

Directions:
1. Add all ingredients except milk, cheese, and yogurt to a crock pot and stir well.
2. Cover and cook on low for 6 hours.
3. Purée the soup using an immersion blender until smooth.
4. Add cheese, milk, and yogurt and blend until smooth and creamy.
5. Season with pepper and salt.
6. Serve and enjoy.

Nutrition: Calories 281 Fat 20 g Carbohydrates 14.4 g Sugar 6.9 g Protein 13.1 g Cholesterol 32 mg

346. Squash Soup

Preparation Time: 10 minutes
Cooking Time: 8 hours
Servings: 6
Ingredients:

- 2 lb butternut squash, peeled, chopped into chunks
- 1 tsp ginger, minced

- 1/4 tsp cinnamon
- 1 Tbsp curry powder
- 2 bay leaves
- 1 tsp black pepper
- 1/2 cup heavy cream
- 2 cups chicken stock
- 1 Tbsp garlic, minced
- 2 carrots, cut into chunks
- 2 apples, peeled, cored and diced
- 1 large onion, diced
- 1 tsp salt

Directions:
1. Spray a crock pot inside with cooking spray.
2. Add all ingredients except cream to the crock pot and stir well.
3. Cover and cook on low for 8 hours.
4. Purée the soup using an immersion blender until smooth and creamy.
5. Stir in heavy cream and season soup with pepper and salt.
6. Serve and enjoy.

Nutrition: Calories 170 Fat 4.4 g Carbohydrates 34.4 g Sugar 13.4g Protein 2.9 g Cholesterol 14 mg

347. Herb Tomato Soup

Preparation Time: 10 minutes
Cooking Time: 6 hours
Servings: 8
Ingredients:

- 55 oz can tomatoes, diced
- 1/2 onion, minced
- 2 cups chicken stock
- 1 cup half and half
- 4 Tbsp butter
- 1 bay leaf
- 1/2 tsp black pepper
- 1/2 tsp garlic powder
- 1 tsp oregano
- 1 tsp dried thyme
- 1 cup carrots, diced
- 1/4 tsp black pepper
- 1/2 tsp salt

Directions:
1. Add all ingredients to a crock pot and stir well.
2. Cover and cook on low for 6 hours.
3. Discard bay leaf and purée the soup using an immersion blender until smooth.
4. Serve and enjoy.

Nutrition: Calories 145 Fat 9.4 g Carbohydrates 13.9 g Sugar 7.9 g Protein 3.2 g Cholesterol 26 mg

348. Easy Beef Mushroom Stew

Preparation Time: 10 minutes
Cooking Time: 8 hours
Servings: 8
Ingredients:

- 2 lb stewing beef, cubed
- 1 packet dry onion soup mix

- 4 oz can mushrooms, sliced
- 14 oz can cream of mushroom soup
- 1/2 cup water
- 1/4 tsp black pepper
- 1/2 tsp salt

Directions:
1. Spray a crock pot inside with cooking spray.
2. Add all ingredients into the crock pot and stir well.
3. Cover and cook on low for 8 hours.
4. Stir well and serve.

Nutrition: Calories 237 Fat 8.5 g Carbohydrates 2.7 g Sugar 0.4 g Protein 35.1 g Cholesterol 101 mg

349. Lamb Stew

Preparation Time: 10 minutes
Cooking Time: 8 hours
Servings: 2
Ingredients:

- 1/2 lb lean lamb, boneless and cubed
- 2 Tbsp lemon juice
- 1/2 onion, chopped
- 2 garlic cloves, minced
- 2 fresh thyme sprigs
- 1/4 tsp turmeric
- 1/4 cup green olives, sliced
- 1/2 tsp black pepper
- 1/4 tsp salt

Directions:
1. Add all ingredients to a crock pot and stir well.
2. Cover and cook on low for 8 hours.
3. Stir well and serve.

Nutrition: Calories 297 Fat 20.3 g Carbohydrates 5.4 g Sugar 1.5 g Protein 21 g Cholesterol 80 mg

350. Vegetable Chicken Soup

Preparation Time: 10 minutes
Cooking Time: 6 hours
Servings: 6
Ingredients:

- 4 cups chicken, boneless, skinless, cooked and diced
- 4 tsp garlic, minced
- 2/3 cups onion, diced
- 1 1/2 cups carrot, diced
- 6 cups chicken stock
- 2 Tbsp lime juice
- 1/4 cup jalapeño pepper, diced
- 1/2 cup tomatoes, diced
- 1/2 cup fresh cilantro, chopped
- 1 tsp chili powder
- 1 Tbsp cumin
- 1 3/4 cups tomato juice
- 2 tsp sea salt

Directions:
1. Add all ingredients to a crock pot and stir well.
2. Cover and cook on low for 6 hours.
3. Stir well and serve.

Nutrition: Calories 192 Fat 3.8 g Carbohydrates 9.8 g Sugar 5.7 g Protein 29.2 g Cholesterol 72 mg

351. Vegan Cream Soup with Avocado & Zucchini

Preparation Time: 15 minutes
Cooking Time: 20 minutes
Servings: 2
Ingredients:

- 3 tsp vegetable oil
- 1 leek, chopped
- 1 rutabaga, sliced
- 3 cups zucchinis, chopped
- 1 avocado, chopped
- Salt and black pepper to taste
- 4 cups vegetable broth
- 2 tbsp fresh mint, chopped

Directions:
1. In a pot, sauté leek, zucchini, and rutabaga in warm oil for about 7-10 minutes. Season with black pepper and salt. Pour in broth and bring to a boil. Lower the heat and simmer for 20 minutes.
2. Lift from the heat. In batches, add the soup and avocado to a blender. Blend until creamy and smooth. Serve in bowls topped with fresh mint.

Nutrition: Calories 378 Fat: 24.5g, Net Carbs: 9.3g, Protein: 8.2g

352. Chinese Tofu Soup

Preparation Time: 5 minutes
Cooking Time: 10 minutes
Servings: 2
Ingredients:

- 2 cups chicken stock
- 1 tbsp soy sauce, sugar-free
- 2 spring onions, sliced
- 1 tsp sesame oil, softened
- 2 eggs, beaten
- 1-inch piece ginger, grated
- Salt and black ground, to taste
- ½ pound extra-firm tofu, cubed
- A handful of fresh cilantro, chopped

Directions:
1. Boil in a pan over medium heat, soy sauce, chicken stock and sesame oil. Place in eggs as you whisk to incorporate completely. Change heat to low and add salt, spring onions, black pepper and ginger; cook for 5 minutes. Place in tofu and simmer for 1 to 2 minutes.
2. Divide into soup bowls and serve sprinkled with fresh cilantro.

Nutrition: Calories 163; Fat: 10g, Net Carbs: 2.4g, Protein: 14.5g

353. Awesome Chicken Enchilada Soup

Preparation Time: 20 minutes
Cooking Time: 30 minutes
Servings: 4
Ingredients:

- 2 tbsp coconut oil

- 1 lb boneless, skinless chicken thighs
- ¾ cup red enchilada sauce, sugar-free
- ¼ cup water
- ¼ cup onion, chopped
- 3 oz canned diced green chilis
- 1 avocado, sliced
- 1 cup cheddar cheese, shredded
- ¼ cup pickled jalapeños, chopped
- ½ cup sour cream
- 1 tomato, diced

Directions:

1. Put a large pan over medium heat. Add coconut oil and warm. Place in the chicken and cook until browned on the outside. Stir in onion, chillis, water, and enchilada sauce, then close with a lid.
2. Allow simmering for 20 minutes until the chicken is cooked through.
3. Spoon the soup on a serving bowl and top with the sauce, cheese, sour cream, tomato, and avocado.

Nutrition: Calories: 643, Fat: 44.2g, Net Carbs: 9.7g, Protein: 45.8g

354. Curried Shrimp & Green Bean Soup

Preparation Time: 10 minutes
Cooking Time: 10 minutes
Servings: 4
Ingredients:

- 1 onion, chopped
- 2 tbsp red curry paste
- 2 tbsp butter
- 1-pound jumbo shrimp, peeled and deveined
- 2 tsp ginger-garlic puree
- 1 cup coconut milk
- Salt and chili pepper to taste
- 1 bunch green beans, halved
- 1 tbsp cilantro, chopped

Directions:

1. Add the shrimp to melted butter in a saucepan over medium heat, season with salt and pepper, and cook until they are opaque, 2 to 3 minutes. Remove to a plate. Add in the ginger-garlic puree, onion, and red curry paste and sauté for 2 minutes until fragrant.
2. Stir in the coconut milk; add the shrimp, salt, chili pepper, and green beans. Cook for 4 minutes. Reduce the heat to a simmer and cook an additional 3 minutes, occasionally stirring. Adjust taste with salt, fetch soup into serving bowls, and serve sprinkled with cilantro.

Nutrition: Calories 351, Fat 32.4g, Net Carbs 3.2g, Protein 7.7g

355. Spinach & Basil Chicken Soup

Preparation Time: 5 minutes
Cooking Time: 10 minutes
Servings: 4
Ingredients:

- 1 cup spinach

- 2 cups cooked and shredded chicken
- 4 cups chicken broth
- 1 cup cheddar cheese, shredded
- 4 ounces' cream cheese
- ½ tsp chili powder
- ½ tsp ground cumin
- ½ tsp fresh parsley, chopped
- Salt and black pepper, to taste

Directions:

1. In a pot, add the chicken broth and spinach, bring to a boil and cook for 5-8 minutes. Transfer to a food processor, add in the cream cheese and pulse until smooth. Return the mixture to a pot and place over medium heat. Cook until hot, but do not bring to a boil.
2. Add chicken, chili powder, and cumin and cook for about 3-5 minutes, or until it is heated through.
3. Stir in cheddar cheese and season with salt and pepper. Serve hot in bowls sprinkled with parsley.

Nutrition: Calories 351, Fat: 22.4g, Net Carbs: 4.3g, Protein: 21.6g

356. Sausage & Turnip Soup

Preparation Time: 20 minutes
Cooking Time: 20 minutes
Servings: 4
Ingredients:

- 3 turnips, chopped
- 2 celery sticks, chopped
- 2 tbsp butter
- 1 tbsp olive oil
- 1 pork sausage, sliced
- 2 cups vegetable broth
- ½ cup sour cream
- 3 green onions, chopped
- 2 cups water
- Salt and black pepper, to taste

Directions:

1. Sauté the green onions in melted butter over medium heat until soft and golden, about 3-4 minutes. Add celery and turnip, and cook for another 5 minutes. Pour over the vegetable broth and water over.
2. Bring to a boil, simmer covered, and cook for about 20 minutes until the vegetables are tender. Remove from heat. Puree the soup with a hand blender until smooth. Add sour cream and adjust the seasoning. Warm the olive oil in a skillet. Add the pork sausage and cook for 5 minutes. Serve the soup in deep bowls topped with pork sausage.

Nutrition: Calories 275, Fat: 23.1g, Net Carbs: 6.4g, Protein: 7.4g

357. Mushroom Cream Soup with Herbs

Preparation Time: 10 minutes
Cooking Time: 15 minutes
Servings: 4
Ingredients:

- 1 onion, chopped
- ½ cup crème fraiche
- ¼ cup butter
- 12 oz white mushrooms, chopped
- 1 tsp thyme leaves, chopped
- 1 tsp parsley leaves, chopped
- 1 tsp cilantro leaves, chopped
- 2 garlic cloves, minced
- 4 cups vegetable broth
- Salt and black pepper, to taste

Directions:

1. Add butter, onion and garlic to a large pot over high heat and cook for 3 minutes until tender. Add mushrooms, salt and pepper, and cook for 10 minutes. Pour in the broth and bring to a boil.
2. Reduce the heat and simmer for 10 minutes. Puree the soup with a hand blender until smooth. Stir in crème fraiche. Garnish with herbs before serving.

Nutrition: Calories 213 Fat: 18g Net Carbs: 4.1g Protein: 3.1g

358. **Broccoli & Spinach Soup**

Preparation Time: 5 minutes
Cooking Time: 20 minutes
Servings: 4
Ingredients:

- 2 tbsp butter
- 1 onion, chopped
- 1 garlic clove, minced
- 2 heads broccoli, cut in florets
- 2 stalks celery, chopped
- 4 cups vegetable broth
- 1 cup baby spinach
- Salt and black pepper to taste
- 1 tbsp basil, chopped
- Parmesan cheese, shaved to serve

Directions:

1. Melt the butter in a saucepan over medium heat. Sauté the garlic and onion for 3 minutes until softened. Mix in the broccoli and celery, and cook for 4 minutes until slightly tender. Pour in the broth, bring to a boil, then reduce the heat to medium-low and simmer covered for about 5 minutes.
2. Drop in the spinach to wilt, adjust the seasonings, and cook for 4 minutes. Ladle soup into serving bowls. Serve with a sprinkle of grated Parmesan cheese and chopped basil.

Nutrition: Calories 123 Fat 11g Net Carbs 3.2g Protein 1.8g

359. **Cheese Cream Soup with Chicken & Cilantro**

Preparation Time: 5 minutes
Cooking Time: 10 minutes
Servings: 4
Ingredients:

- 1 carrot, chopped
- 1 onion, chopped

- 2 cups cooked and shredded chicken
- 3 tbsp butter
- 4 cups chicken broth
- 2 tbsp cilantro, chopped
- 1/3 cup buffalo sauce
- ½ cup cream cheese
- Salt and black pepper, to taste

Directions:

1. In a skillet over medium heat, warm butter and sauté carrot and onion until tender, about 5 minutes.
2. Add to a food processor and blend with buffalo sauce and cream cheese, until smooth. Transfer to a pot, add chicken broth and heat until hot but do not bring to a boil. Stir in chicken, salt, pepper and cook until heated through. When ready, remove to soup bowls and serve garnished with cilantro.

Nutrition: Calories 487, Fat: 41g, Net Carbs: 7.2g, Protein: 16.3g

360. **Thick Creamy Broccoli Cheese Soup**

Preparation Time: 10 minutes
Cooking Time: 10 minutes
Servings: 4
Ingredients:

- 1 tbsp olive oil
- 2 tbsp peanut butter
- ¾ cup heavy cream
- 1 onion, diced
- 1 garlic, minced
- 4 cups chopped broccoli
- 4 cups veggie broth
- 2 ¾ cups cheddar cheese, grated
- ¼ cup cheddar cheese to garnish
- Salt and black pepper, to taste
- ½ bunch fresh mint, chopped

Directions:

1. Warm olive oil and peanut butter in a pot over medium heat. Sauté onion and garlic for 3 minutes or until tender, stirring occasionally. Season with salt and black pepper. Add the broth and broccoli and bring to a boil.
2. Reduce the heat and simmer for 10 minutes. Puree the soup with a hand blender until smooth. Add in the cheese and cook about 1 minute. Stir in the heavy cream. Serve in bowls with the reserved grated cheddar cheese and sprinkled with fresh mint.

Nutrition: Calories 552, Fat: 49.5g, Net Carbs: 6.9g, Protein: 25g

361. **Vegetarian Split Pea Soup in a Crock Pot**

Preparation Time: 10 minutes
Cooking Time: 10 minutes
Servings: 8
Ingredients:

- 2 chopped ribs celery

- 2 cubes low-sodium bouillon
- 8 c. water
- 2 c. uncooked green split peas
- 3 bay leaves
- 2 carrots
- 2 chopped potatoes
- Pepper and salt

Directions:

1. In your Crock-Pot, put the bouillon cubes, split peas, and water. Stir a bit to break up the bouillon cubes.
2. Next, add the chopped potatoes, celery, and carrots followed with bay leaves.
3. Stir to combine well.
4. Cover and cook for at least 4 hours on your Crock-Pot's low setting or until the green split peas are soft.
5. Add a bit salt and pepper as needed.
6. Before serving, remove the bay leaves and enjoy.

Nutrition: Calories: 149, Fat:1 g, Carbs:30 g, Protein:7 g, Sugars:3 g, Sodium:732 mg

362. Rhubarb Stew

Preparation Time: 5 minutes
Cooking Time: 10 minutes
Servings: 3
Ingredients:

- 1 tsp. grated lemon zest
- 1 ½ c. coconut sugar
- Juice of 1 lemon
- 1 ½ c. water
- 4 ½ c. roughly chopped rhubarbs

Directions:

1. In a pan, combine the rhubarb while using water, fresh lemon juice, lemon zest and coconut sugar, toss, bring using a simmer over medium heat, cook for 5 minutes, and divide into bowls and serve cold.
2. Enjoy!

Nutrition: Calories: 108, Fat:1 g, Carbs:8 g, Protein:5 g, Sugars:2 g, Sodium:0 mg

363. Tofu Soup

Preparation Time: 5 minutes
Cooking Time: 10 minutes
Servings: 8
Ingredients:

- 1 lb. cubed extra-firm tofu
- 3 diced medium carrots
- 8 c. low-sodium vegetable broth
- ½ tsp. freshly ground white pepper
- 8 minced garlic cloves
- 6 sliced and divided scallions
- 4 oz. sliced mushrooms
- 1-inch minced fresh ginger piece

Directions:

1. Pour the broth into a stockpot. Add all of the ingredients except for the tofu and last 2 scallions. Bring to a boil over high heat.

2. Once boiling, add the tofu. Reduce heat to low, cover, and simmer for 5 minutes.
3. Remove from heat, ladle soup into bowls, and garnish with the remaining sliced scallions. Serve immediately.

Nutrition: Calories: 91, Fat:3 g, Carbs:8 g, Protein:6 g, Sugars:4 g, Sodium:900 mg

364. Easy Beef Stew

Preparation Time: 5 minutes
Cooking Time: 5 minutes
Servings: 6
Ingredients:

- 1 shredded green cabbage head
- 4 chopped carrots
- 2 ½ lbs. non-fat beef brisket
- 3 chopped garlic cloves
- Black pepper
- 2 bay leaves
- 4 c. low-sodium beef stock

Directions:

1. Put the beef brisket in a pot, add stock, pepper, garlic and bay leaves, provide your simmer over medium heat and cook for an hour.
2. Add carrots and cabbage, stir, cook for a half-hour more, divide into bowls and serve for lunch.
3. Enjoy!

Nutrition: Calories: 271, Fat:8 g,Carbs:16 g, Protein:9 g, Sugars:3.4 g, Sodium:760 mg

365. Zucchini-Basil Soup

Preparation Time: 20 minutes
Cooking Time: 10 minutes
Servings: 5
Ingredients:

- 1/3 c. packed basil leaves
- ¾ c. chopped onion
- ¼ c. olive oil
- 2 lbs. trimmed and sliced zucchini
- 2 chopped garlic cloves
- 4 c. divided water

Directions:

1. Peel and julienne the skin from half of zucchini; toss with 1/2 teaspoon salt and drain in a sieve until wilted, at least 20 minutes. Coarsely chop remaining zucchini.
2. Cook onion and garlic in oil in a saucepan over medium-low heat, stirring occasionally, until onions are translucent. Add chopped zucchini and 1 teaspoon salt and cook, stirring occasionally.
3. Add 3 cups water and simmer with the lid ajar until tender. Pour the soup in a blender and purée soup with basil.
4. Bring remaining cup water to a boil in a small saucepan and blanch julienned zucchini. Drain.
5. Top soup with julienned zucchini. Season soup with salt and pepper and serve.

Nutrition: Calories: 169.3, Fat:13.7 g, Carbs:12 g, Protein:2 g,Sugars:3.8 g, Sodium:8 mg

366. <u>Black Bean Soup</u>

Preparation Time: 10 minutes
Cooking Time: 10 minutes
Servings: 4
Ingredients:

- 1 tsp. cinnamon powder
- 32 oz. low-sodium chicken stock
- 1 chopped yellow onion
- 1 chopped sweet potato
- 38 oz. no-salt-added, drained and rinsed canned black beans
- 2 tsps. organic olive oil

Directions:

1. Heat up a pot using the oil over medium heat, add onion and cinnamon, stir and cook for 6 minutes.
2. Add black beans, stock and sweet potato, stir, cook for 14 minutes, puree utilizing an immersion blender, divide into bowls and serve for lunch.
3. Enjoy!

Nutrition: Calories: 221, Fat:3 g,Carbs:15 g, Protein:7 g, Sugars:4 g, Sodium:511 mg

367. <u>Chicken and Dill Soup</u>

Preparation Time: 10 minutes
Cooking Time: 10 minutes
Servings: 6
Ingredients:

- 1 c. chopped yellow onion
- 1 whole chicken
- 1 lb. sliced carrots
- 6 c. low-sodium veggie stock
- ¼ tsp. black pepper and salt
- ½ c. chopped red onion
- 2 tsps. chopped dill

Directions:

1. Put chicken in a pot, add water to pay for, give your boil over medium heat, cook first hour, transfer to a cutting board, discard bones, shred the meat, strain the soup, get it back on the pot, heat it over medium heat and add the chicken.
2. Also add the carrots, yellow onion, red onion, a pinch of salt, black pepper and also the dill, cook for fifteen minutes, ladle into bowls and serve.
3. Enjoy!

Nutrition: Calories: 202, Fat:6 g, Carbs:8 g, Protein:12 g, Sugars:6 g, Sodium:514 mg

368. <u>Cherry Stew</u>

Preparation Time: 10 minutes
Cooking Time: 10 minutes
Servings: 6
Ingredients:

- 2 c. water
- ½ c. powered cocoa
- ¼ c. coconut sugar
- 1 lb. pitted cherries

Directions:

1. In a pan, combine the cherries with all the water, sugar plus the hot chocolate mix, stir, cook over

medium heat for ten minutes, divide into bowls and serve cold.
2. Enjoy!

Nutrition: Calories: 207, Fat:1 g, Carbs:8 g, Protein:6 g, Sugars:27 g, Sodium:19 mg

369. <u>Sirloin Carrot Soup</u>

Preparation Time: 10 minutes
Cooking Time: 10 minutes
Servings: 6
Ingredients:

- 1 lb. chopped carrots and celery mix
- 32 oz. low-sodium beef stock
- 1/3 c. whole-wheat flour
- 1 lb. ground beef sirloin
- 1 tbsp. olive oil
- 1 chopped yellow onion

Directions:

1. Heat up the olive oil in a saucepan over medium-high flame; add the beef and the flour.
2. Stir well and cook to brown for 4-5 minutes.
3. Add the celery, onion, carrots, and stock; stir and bring to a simmer.
4. Turn down the heat to low and cook for 12-15 minutes.
5. Serve warm.

Nutrition: Calories: 140, Fat: 4.5 g,Carbs: 16 g, Protein: 9 g, Sugars: 3 g, Sodium:670 mg

370. <u>Easy Wonton Soup</u>

Preparation Time: 10 minutes
Cooking Time: 20 minutes
Servings: 6
Ingredients:

- 4 sliced scallions
- ¼ tsp. ground white pepper
- 2 c. sliced fresh mushrooms
- 4 minced garlic cloves
- 6 oz. dry whole-grain yolk-free egg noodles
- ½ lb. lean ground pork
- 1 tbsp. minced fresh ginger
- 8 c. low-sodium chicken broth

Directions:

1. Place a stockpot over medium heat. Add the ground pork, ginger, and garlic and sauté for 5 minutes. Drain any excess fat, then return to stovetop.
2. Add the broth and bring to a boil. Once boiling, stir in the mushrooms, noodles, and white pepper. Cover and simmer for 10 minutes.
3. Remove pot from heat. Stir in the scallions and serve immediately.

Nutrition: Calories: 143, Fat:4 g, Carbs:14 g, Protein:12 g, Sugars:0.8 g, Sodium:901 mg

371. <u>Beef & Mushroom Barley Soup</u>

Preparation Time: 10 minutes
Cooking Time: 1 hour and 20 minutes
Servings: 6

Ingredients:

- ½ cup of pearl barley
- 1 cup of water
- 4 cups of low-sodium beef broth
- ½ teaspoon thyme, dried
- 6 garlic cloves, minced
- 3 celery stalks, chopped
- 1 onion, chopped
- 2 carrots, chopped
- 8-ounces of mushrooms, sliced
- 1 tablespoon extra-virgin olive oil
- ¼ teaspoon freshly ground black pepper
- 1 lb. Of beef stew meat, cubed

Directions:

1. Season your meat with salt and pepper.
2. Heat the oil in an Instant Pot over high heat. Add the beef and brown, then remove meat and set aside.
3. Add your mushrooms to the pot and cook for about 1 to 2 minutes or until they begin to soften. Remove the mushrooms from pot and set them aside along with the meat.
4. Add your carrots, celery, and onions into the pot. Sauté vegetables for about 4 minutes or until they begin to soften. Add your garlic into pot and cook until fragrant.
5. Place the meat and mushrooms back into the pot, then add the beef broth, thyme, and water. Set your pot pressure to high and cook for 15 minutes. Allow the pressure to release naturally.
6. Open your Instant Pot and add the barley. Use the slow cooker function on the pot, with the lid having vent open, then continue cooking for an additional hour or until your barley is cooked and tender. Serve and enjoy!

Nutrition: Carbs per serving: 19g

372. Chicken Tortilla Soup

Preparation Time: 10 minutes
Cooking Time: 35 minutes
Servings: 4
Ingredients:

- ¼ cup of cheddar cheese, shredded, for garnish
- fresh cilantro, minced, for garnish
- juice of 1 lime
- nonstick cooking spray
- 2 (6-inch) corn tortillas, sliced into thin slices
- ½ teaspoon salt
- 1 Roma tomato, diced
- 4 cups of low-sodium chicken broth
- 2 boneless, skinless chicken breasts
- 1 jalapeno pepper, diced
- 1 garlic clove, minced
- 1 onion, thinly sliced
- 1 tablespoon extra-virgin olive oil

Directions:

1. Heat your oil in a pot over medium-high heat. Add your onions and cook for 3-5 minutes or until they

begin to soften. Add your garlic and jalapeno, then cook for an additional minute.

2. Add your chicken, tomato, chicken broth, and salt to the pot and bring to a boil. Reduce the heat setting to medium and simmer for about 20 minutes or until the chicken breasts are cooked through. Remove your chicken from the pot and set aside.
3. Preheat a broiler to high.
4. Spray the tortilla strips with some nonstick cooking spray and toss to coat. Place your tortilla strips in a single layer on a baking sheet, then broil for 3-5 minutes, flipping them once, until crisp.
5. Once your chicken has cooled, shred it using two forks and return to pot.
6. Season the soup with the lime juice. Serve hot, garnished with cheese, cilantro, and tortilla strips and enjoy!

Nutrition: Carbs per serving: 13g

373. Thai Peanut, Carrot, & Shrimp Soup

Preparation Time: 10 minutes
Cooking Time: 10 minutes
Servings: 4
Ingredients:

- 3 garlic cloves, minced
- ½ onion, sliced
- 1 tablespoon Thai red curry paste
- 1 tablespoon coconut oil
- fresh cilantro, minced, for garnish
- ½ pound shrimp, peeled and deveined
- ½ cup unsweetened plain almond milk
- 4 cups of low-sodium vegetable broth
- ½ cup whole unsalted peanuts
- 2 cups carrots, chopped

Directions:

1. In a pan, heat your oil over medium-high heat until shimmering.
2. Add your curry paste to the pan and cook continually stirring for about 1 minute. Add the garlic, onion, and carrots, along with peanuts to the pan. Continue cooking for 3 minutes or until your onion begins to soften.
3. Add your broth and bring to a boil. Reduce heat to a low setting and simmer for 6 minutes or until carrots are tender.
4. Use your immersion blender to puree your soup until smooth and return to pot. With heat setting on low, add the almond milk and stir to combine. Add your shrimp to the pot and cook for 3 minutes or until cooked.
5. Garnish soup with cilantro, then serve and enjoy!

Nutrition: Carbs per serving: 17g

374. Curried Carrot Soup

Preparation Time: 10 minutes
Cooking Time: 5 minutes
Servings: 6
Ingredients:

- 2 celery stalks, chopped
- 1 small onion, chopped
- 1 tablespoon extra-virgin olive oil
- 1 tablespoon fresh cilantro, chopped
- ¼ teaspoon freshly ground black pepper
- 1 cup of canned coconut milk
- ¼ teaspoon salt
- 4 cups of low-sodium vegetable broth
- 6 medium carrots, roughly chopped
- 1 teaspoon fresh ginger, minced
- 1 teaspoon ground cumin
- 1 ½ teaspoon curry powder

Directions:

1. Heat your Instant Pot to high setting and add the olive oil.
2. Sauté your celery and onion for 3 minutes. Add the curry powder, ginger, and cumin to the pot and cook for about 30 seconds.
3. Add the carrots, vegetable broth, and salt to your pot. Close pot and seal and set on high for 5 minutes. Allow the pressure to release naturally.
4. Pure your soup in batches in a blender jar and transfer back into the pot.
5. Stir in the coconut milk along with pepper and heat through. Top soup with cilantro, then serve and enjoy!

Nutrition: Carbs per serving: 13g

375. **Summer Squash Soup with Crispy Chickpeas**

Preparation Time: 10 minutes
Cooking Time: 20 minutes
Servings: 4
Ingredients:

- ¼ teaspoon smoked paprika
- 1 teaspoon extra-virgin olive oil, plus one tablespoon
- 1 (15-ounce) can low-sodium chickpeas, drained and rinsed
- 2 tablespoons plain low-fat Greek yogurt
- freshly ground black pepper
- 3 garlic cloves, minced
- ½ onion, diced
- 3 cups of low-sodium vegetable broth
- 3 medium zucchinis, coarsely chopped
- pinch of sea salt, plus ½ teaspoon

Directions:

1. Preheat your oven to 425° Fahrenheit. Line a baking sheet with some parchment paper.
2. In a mixing bowl, toss your chickpeas with one teaspoon of olive oil, the smoked paprika, and a pinch of sea salt. Transfer your mixture to the baking sheet, then roast until crispy for about 20 minutes, stirring once. Set aside.
3. In a pot, heat the remaining 1 tablespoon of oil over medium heat.
4. Add your zucchini, onion, broth, and garlic to the pot and bring to a boil. Lower the heat to simmer,

then cook until the onion and zucchini are tender, for about 20 minutes.

5. In a blender jar, puree your soup, then return it to the pot.
6. Add the yogurt, and the remaining ½ teaspoon of sea salt, and pepper, then stir well. Serve topped with roasted chickpeas and enjoy!

Nutrition: Carbs per serving: 24g

376. **Cream Zucchini Soup**

Preparation Time: 8 minutes
Cooking Time: 8 minutes
Servings: 4
Ingredients:

- 2 cups vegetable stock
- 2 garlic cloves, crushed
- 1 tablespoon butter
- 4 (preferably medium size) zucchinis, peeled and chopped
- 1 small onion, chopped
- 2 cups heavy cream
- 1/2 teaspoon dried oregano, (finely ground)
- 1/2 teaspoon black pepper, (finely ground)
- 1 teaspoon dried parsley, (finely ground)
- 1 teaspoon of sea salt
- Lemon juice (optional)

Directions:

1. Arrange Instant Pot over a dry platform in your kitchen. Open its top lid and switch it on.
2. Find and press "SAUTE" cooking function; add the butter in it and allow it to melt.
3. In the pot, add the onions, zucchini, garlic; cook (while stirring) until turns translucent and softened for around 2-3 minutes.
4. Add the vegetable broth and sprinkle with salt, oregano, pepper, and parsley; gently stir to mix well.
5. Close the lid to create a locked chamber; make sure that safety valve is in locking position.
6. Find and press "MANUAL" cooking function; timer to 5 minutes with default "HIGH" pressure mode.
7. Allow the pressure to build to cook the ingredients.
8. After cooking time is over press "CANCEL" setting. Find and press "QPR" cooking function. This setting is for quick release of inside pressure.
9. Slowly open the lid, take out the cooked in serving plates or serving bowls, and enjoy the keto . Top with some lemon juice.

Nutrition: Calories - 264 Fat: 26g Saturated Fat: 7g Trans Fat: 0g Carbohydrates: 11g Fiber: 3g Sodium: 564mg Protein: 4g

377. **Coconut Chicken Soup**

Preparation Time: 8 minutes
Cooking Time: 18 minutes
Servings: 4
Ingredients:

- 4 cloves of garlic, minced
- 1-pound chicken breasts, skin-on

- 4 cups of water
- 2 tablespoons olive oil
- 1 onion, diced
- 1 cup of coconut milk
- (finely ground) black pepper and salt as per taste preference
- 2 tablespoons sesame oil

Directions:

1. Arrange Instant Pot over a dry platform in your kitchen. Open its top lid and switch it on.
2. Find and press "SAUTE" cooking function; add the oil in it and allow it to heat.
3. In the pot, add the onions, garlic; cook (while stirring) until turns translucent and softened for around 1-2 minutes.
4. Stir in the chicken breasts; stir, and cook for 2 more minutes.
5. Pour in water and coconut milk — season to taste.
6. Close the lid to create a locked chamber; make sure that safety valve is in locking position.
7. Find and press "MANUAL" cooking function; timer to 15 minutes with default "HIGH" pressure mode.
8. Allow the pressure to build to cook the ingredients.
9. After cooking time is over press "CANCEL" setting. Find and press "NPR" cooking function. This setting is for the natural release of inside pressure and it takes around 10 minutes to slowly release pressure.
10. Slowly open the lid, Drizzle with sesame oil on top.
11. Take out the cooked in serving plates or serving bowls and enjoy the keto.

Nutrition: Calories - 328 Fat: 31g Saturated Fat: 6g Trans Fat: 0g Carbohydrates: 6g Fiber: 4g Sodium: 76mg Protein: 21g

378. Chicken Bacon Soup

Preparation Time: 10 minutes
Cooking Time: 40 minutes
Servings: 4
Ingredients:

- 6 boneless, skinless chicken thighs, make cubes
- ½ cup chopped celery
- 4 minced garlic cloves
- 6-ounce mushrooms, sliced
- ½ cup chopped onion
- 8-ounce softened cream cheese
- ¼ cup softened butter
- 1 teaspoon dried thyme
- Salt and (finely ground) black pepper, as per taste preference
- 2 cups chopped spinach
- 8 ounces cooked bacon slices, chopped
- 3 cups (preferably homemade) chicken broth
- 1 cup heavy cream

Directions:

1. Arrange Instant Pot over a dry platform in your kitchen. Open its top lid and switch it on.

2. Add the ingredients except for the cream, spinach, and bacon; gently stir to mix well.
3. Close the lid to create a locked chamber; make sure that safety valve is in locking position.
4. Find and press "SOUP" cooking function; timer to 30 minutes with default "HIGH" pressure mode.
5. Allow the pressure to build to cook the ingredients.
6. After cooking time is over press "CANCEL" setting. Find and press "NPR" cooking function. This setting is for the natural release of inside pressure and it takes around 10 minutes to slowly release pressure.
7. Slowly open the lid, stir in cream and spinach.
8. Take out the cooked in serving plates or serving bowls and enjoy the keto. Top with the bacon.

Nutrition: Calories - 456 Fat: 38g Saturated Fat: 13g Trans Fat: 0g Carbohydrates: 7g Fiber: 1g Sodium: 742mg Protein: 23g

379. Cream Pepper Stew

Preparation Time: 20 minutes
Cooking Time: 10 min.
Servings: 4
Ingredients:

- 1 (preferably medium size) celery stalk, chopped
- 1 (preferably medium size) yellow bell pepper, chopped
- 1 (preferably medium size) green bell pepper, chopped
- 2 large red bell peppers, chopped
- 1 small red onion, chopped
- 2 tablespoons butter
- 1/2 cup cream cheese, full-fat
- 1/4 teaspoon dried thyme, (finely ground)
- 1/2 teaspoon black pepper, (finely ground)
- 1 teaspoon dried parsley, (finely ground)
- 1 teaspoon salt
- 2 cups vegetable stock
- 1 cup heavy cream

Directions:

1. Arrange Instant Pot over a dry platform in your kitchen. Open its top lid and switch it on.
2. Find and press "SAUTE" cooking function; add the butter in it and allow it to heat.
3. In the pot, add the onions, bell pepper, and celery; cook (while stirring) until turns translucent and softened for around 3-4 minutes.
4. Pour in the vegetable stock and heavy cream — season with salt, pepper, parsley, and thyme.
5. Close the lid to create a locked chamber; make sure that safety valve is in locking position.
6. Find and press "MANUAL" cooking function; timer to 6 minutes with default "HIGH" pressure mode.
7. Allow the pressure to build to cook the ingredients.
8. After cooking time is over press "CANCEL" setting. Find and press "QPR" cooking function. This setting is for quick release of inside pressure.

9. Slowly open the lid, mix in the cream; take out the cooked in serving plates or serving bowls, and enjoy the keto .

Nutrition: Calories - 286 Fat: 27g Saturated Fat: 6g Trans Fat: 0g Carbohydrates: 9g Fiber: 3g Sodium: 523mg Protein: 5g

380. **Ham Asparagus Soup**

Preparation Time: 20 minutes
Cooking Time: 55 min.
Servings: 3-4
Ingredients:

- 5 crushed garlic cloves
- 1 cup chopped ham
- 4 cups (preferably homemade) chicken broth
- 2 pounds trimmed and halved asparagus spears
- 2 tablespoons butter
- 1 chopped yellow onion
- ½ teaspoon dried thyme
- Salt and freshly (finely ground) black pepper, as per taste preference

Directions:

1. Arrange Instant Pot over a dry platform in your kitchen. Open its top lid and switch it on.
2. Find and press "SAUTE" cooking function; add the butter in it and allow it to heat.
3. In the pot, add the onions; cook (while stirring) until turns translucent and softened for around 4-5 minutes.
4. Add the garlic, ham bone and broth; stir, and cook for about 2-3 minutes.
5. Add the other ingredients; gently stir to mix well.
6. Close the lid to create a locked chamber; make sure that safety valve is in locking position.
7. Find and press "SOUP" cooking function; timer to 45 minutes with default "HIGH" pressure mode.
8. Allow the pressure to build to cook the ingredients.
9. After cooking time is over press "CANCEL" setting. Find and press "QPR" cooking function. This setting is for quick release of inside pressure.
10. Slowly open the lid, add the mix in a blender or processor.
11. Blend or process to make a smooth mix. Place the mix in serving bowls and enjoy the keto.

Nutrition: Calories - 146 Fat: 7g Saturated Fat: 3g Trans Fat: 0g Carbohydrates: 5g Fiber: 4g Sodium: 262mg Protein: 10g

381. **Simple Chicken Soup**

Preparation Time: 20 minutes
Cooking Time: 25 minutes
Servings: 4
Ingredients:

- 2 frozen, boneless chicken breasts
- 4 medium-sized potatoes, cut into chunks
- 3 carrots, peeled and cut into chunks
- ½ big onion, diced
- 2 cups chicken stock
- 2 cups water
- Salt and ground black pepper to taste

Directions:

1. In the Instant Pot, combine the chicken breasts, potatoes, carrots, onion, stock, water, salt and pepper to taste.
2. Close and lock the lid. Select MANUAL and cook at HIGH pressure for 25 minutes.
3. Once timer goes off, allow to Naturally Release for 10 minutes, and then release any remaining pressure manually. Uncover the pot.
4. Serve.

Nutrition: Calories 301 Fat 27.2 g Carbohydrates 13.6 g Sugar 6 g Protein 4.9 g Cholesterol 33 mg

382. **Buffalo Chicken Soup**

Preparation Time: 20 minutes
Cooking Time: 30 minutes
Servings: 8
Ingredients:

- 2 chicken breasts, boneless, skinless, frozen or fresh
- 1 clove garlic, chopped
- ¼ cup onion, diced
- ½ cup celery, diced
- 2 tbsp butter
- 1 tbsp ranch dressing mix
- 3 cups chicken broth
- 1/3 cup hot sauce
- 2 cups cheddar cheese, shredded
- 1 cup heavy cream

Directions:

1. In the Instant Pot, combine the chicken breasts, garlic, onion, celery, butter, ranch dressing mix, broth, and hot sauce.
2. Close and lock the lid. Select MANUAL and cook at HIGH pressure for 10 minutes.
3. Once cooking is complete, let the pressure Release Naturally for 10 minutes. Release any remaining steam manually. Uncover the pot.
4. Transfer the chicken to a plate and shred the meat. Return to the pot.
5. Add the cheese and heavy cream. Stir well. Let sit for 5 minutes and serve.

Nutrition: Calories 303 Fat 27.5 g Carbohydrates 13.8 g Sugar 5 g Protein 4.g Cholesterol 33 mg

383. **Beef Borscht Soup**

Preparation Time: 20 minutes
Cooking Time: 30 minutes
Servings: 8
Ingredients:

- 2 lbs ground beef
- 3 beets, peeled and diced
- 2 large carrots, diced
- 3 stalks of celery, diced
- 1 onion, diced
- 2 cloves garlic, diced
- 3 cups shredded cabbage
- 6 cups beef stock
- ½ tbsp thyme
- 1 bay leaf
- Salt and ground black pepper to taste

Directions:

1. Preheat the Instant Pot by selecting SAUTÉ.
2. Add the ground beef and cook, stirring, for 5 minutes, until browned.
3. Combine all the rest ingredients in the Instant Pot and stir to mix. Close and lock the lid.
4. Press the CANCEL button to stop the SAUTÉ function, then select the MANUAL setting and set the cooking time for 15 minutes at HIGH pressure.
5. Once timer goes off, allow to Naturally Release for 10 minutes, then release any remaining pressure manually. Uncover the pot.
6. Let the dish sit for 5-10 minutes and serve.

Nutrition: Calories 301 Fat 27.2 g Carbohydrates 13.6 g Sugar 6 g Protein 3 g Cholesterol 33 mg

384. Beef Barley Soup

Preparation Time: 20 minutes
Cooking Time: 30 minutes
Servings: 8
Ingredients:

- 2 tbsp olive oil
- 2 lbs beef chuck roast, cut into 1½ inch steaks
- Salt and ground black pepper to taste
- 2 onions, chopped
- 4 cloves of garlic, sliced
- 4 large carrots, chopped
- 1 stalk of celery, chopped
- 1 cup pearl barley, rinsed
- 1 bay leaf
- 8 cups chicken stock
- 1 tbsp fish sauce

Directions:

1. Select the SAUTÉ setting on the Instant Pot and heat the oil.
2. Sprinkle the beef with salt and pepper. Put in the pot and brown for about 5 minutes. Turn and brown the other side.
3. Remove the meat from the pot.
4. Add the onion, garlic, carrots, and celery. Stir and sauté for 6 minutes.
5. Return the beef to the pot. Add the pearl barley, bay leaf, chicken stock and fish sauce. Stir well.

6. Close and lock the lid. Press the CANCEL button to reset the cooking program, then press the MANUAL button and set the cooking time for 30 minutes at HIGH pressure.
7. Once cooking is complete, let the pressure Release Naturally for 15 minutes. Release any remaining steam manually. Uncover the pot.
8. Remove cloves garlic, large vegetable chunks and bay leaf.
9. Taste for seasoning and add more salt if needed.

Nutrition: Calories 200 Fat 27.2 g Carbohydrates 13.6 g Sugar 2 g Protein 4.4 g Cholesterol 32 mg

385. Beef and Cabbage Soup

Preparation Time: 20 minutes
Cooking Time: 35 minutes
Servings: 6
Ingredients:

- 2 tbsp coconut oil
- 1 onion, diced
- 1 clove garlic, minced
- 1 lb ground beef
- 14 oz can diced tomatoes, undrained
- 4 cups water
- Salt and ground black pepper to taste
- 1 head cabbage, chopped

Directions:

1. Preheat the Instant Pot by selecting SAUTÉ. Add and heat the oil.
2. Add the onion and garlic and sauté for 2 minutes.
3. Add the beef and cook, stirring, for 2-3 minutes until lightly brown.
4. Pour in the water and tomatoes. Season with salt and pepper, stir well.
5. Press the CANCEL key to stop the SAUTÉ function.
6. Close and lock the lid. Select MANUAL and cook at HIGH pressure for 12 minutes.
7. When the timer goes off, use a Quick Release. Carefully open the lid.
8. Add the cabbage, select SAUTÉ and simmer for 5 minutes.
9. Serve.

Nutrition: Calories 335 Fat 10 g Carbohydrates 13.6 g Sugar 6 g Protein 4.9 g Cholesterol 33 mg

SNACK RECIPES

386. Nori Snack Rolls

Preparation Time: 5 minutes
Cooking Time: 10 minutes
Servings: 4
Ingredients:

- 2 tablespoons almond, cashew, peanut, or other nut butter
- 2 tablespoons tamari, or soy sauce
- 4 standard nori sheets
- 1 mushroom, sliced
- 1 tablespoon pickled ginger
- ½ cup grated carrots

Directions:

1. Preparing the Ingredients.
2. Preheat the oven to 350°F.
3. Mix together the nut butter and tamari until smooth and very thick.
4. Spread a thin line of the tamari mixture on the far end of the nori sheet, from side to side. Lay the mushroom slices, ginger, and carrots in a line at the other end (the end closest to you).
5. Fold the vegetables inside the nori, rolling toward the tahini mixture, which will seal the roll. Repeat to make 4 rolls.
6. Finish and Serve
7. Place on a baking sheet until the rolls are slightly browned and crispy at the ends. Let the rolls cool for a few minutes, then slice each roll into 3 smaller pieces.

Nutrition: Calories: 79 Total fat: 5g Carbs: 6g Fiber: 2g Protein: 4g

387. Risotto Bites

Preparation Time: 15 minutes
Cooking Time: 20 minutes
Servings: 12
Ingredients:

- ½ cup panko bread crumbs
- 1 teaspoon paprika
- 1 teaspoon chipotle powder or ground cayenne pepper
- 1½ cups cold Green Pea Risotto
- Nonstick cooking spray

Directions:

1. Preparing the Ingredients
2. Preheat the oven to 425°F.
3. Line a baking sheet with parchment paper.
4. On a large plate, combine the panko, paprika, and chipotle powder. Set aside.
5. Roll 2 tablespoons of the risotto into a ball.
6. Gently roll in the bread crumbs, and place on the prepared baking sheet. Repeat to make a total of 12 balls.
7. Bake

8. Spritz the tops of the risotto bites with nonstick cooking spray and bake for 15-20 minutes until they begin to brown.
9. Finish and Serve
10. Cool completely before storing in a large airtight container in a single layer (add a piece of parchment paper for a second layer), or in a plastic freezer bag.

Nutrition: Calories: 100 Fat: 2g Protein: 6g Carbohydrates: 17g Fiber: 5g Sugar: 2g Sodium: 165mg

388. Garden Patch Sandwiches On Multigrain Bread

Preparation Time: 15 minutes
Cooking Time: 0 minutes
Servings: 4
Ingredients:

- 1 pound extra-firm tofu, drained and patted dry
- 1 medium red bell pepper, finely chopped
- 1 celery rib, finely chopped
- 3 green onions, minced
- ¼ cup shelled sunflower seeds
- ½ cup vegan mayonnaise, homemade or store-bought
- ½ teaspoon salt
- ½ teaspoon celery salt
- ¼ teaspoon freshly ground black pepper
- 8 slices whole grain bread
- 4 (¼-inch) slices ripe tomato
- 4 lettuce leaves

Directions:

1. Preparing the Ingredients
2. Smash the tofu and place it in a large bowl. Add the bell pepper, celery, green onions, and sunflower seeds. Stir in the mayonnaise, salt, celery salt, and pepper and mix until well combined.
3. Finish and Serve
4. Toast the bread, if desired. Spread the mixture evenly onto 4 slices of the bread.

Nutrition: 166 Cal 15 g Fats 6.5 g Protein 2 g Net Carb 0 g Fiber

389. Garden Salad Wraps

Preparation Time: 15 minutes
Cooking Time: 10 minutes
Servings: 4
Ingredients:

- 6 tablespoons extra-virgin olive oil
- 1-pound extra-firm tofu, drained, patted dry, and cut into ½-inch strips
- 1 tablespoon soy sauce
- ¼ cup apple cider vinegar
- 1 teaspoon yellow or spicy brown mustard
- ½ teaspoon salt
- ¼ teaspoon freshly ground black pepper
- 3 cups shredded romaine lettuce
- 3 ripe Roma tomatoes, finely chopped

- 1 large carrot, shredded
- 1 medium English cucumber, peeled and chopped
- ⅓ cup minced red onion
- ¼ cup sliced pitted green olives
- 4 (10-inch) whole-grain flour tortillas or lavish flatbread

Directions:
1. Preparing the Ingredients
2. Cook the tofu until golden brown in a large skillet with Over medium heat. Sprinkle with soy sauce and set aside to cool.
3. In a small bowl, combine the vinegar, mustard, salt and pepper with the remaining 4 tablespoons oil, stirring to blend well. Set aside.
4. Finish and Serve
5. combine the cucumber, onion, lettuce, tomatoes, carrot, and olives in a large bowl. Pour on the dressing.
6. Put 1 tortilla on a work surface and spread with about one-quarter of the salad. Place a few strips of tofu on the tortilla and roll up tightly. Slice in half.

Nutrition: 191 Cal 16.6 g Fats 9.6 g Protein 0.8 g Net Carb 0.2 g Fiber

390. **Black Sesame Wonton Chips**

Preparation Time: 5 minutes
Cooking Time: 5 minutes
Servings: 24
Ingredients:

- 12 Vegan Wonton Wrappers
- Toasted sesame oil
- ⅓ cup black sesame seeds
- Salt

Directions:
1. Preparing the Ingredients
2. Preheat the oven to 450°F. Arrange the wonton wrapper in a single layer on the prepared baking sheet. and cut it in half crosswise and brush them with sesame oil.
3. Sprinkle wonton wrappers with the sesame seeds and salt.
4. Bake
5. Bake until crisp and golden brown.
6. Finish and Serve
7. Cool completely before serving. These are best eaten on the day they are made but once cooled, they can be covered and stored at room temperature for 1-2 days.

Nutrition: Fat: 1.2 g Protein: 3.6 g Carbohydrates: 11.6 g

391. **Marinated Mushroom Wraps**

Preparation Time: 15 minutes
Cooking Time: 0 minutes
Servings: 2
Ingredients:

- 3 tablespoons soy sauce
- 3 tablespoons fresh lemon juice
- 1½ tablespoons toasted sesame oil
- 2 portobello mushroom caps, cut into 1/4-inch strips

- 1 ripe Hass avocado, pitted and peeled
- 2 (10-inch) whole-grain flour tortillas
- 2 cups fresh baby spinach leaves
- 1 medium red bell pepper, cut into ¼ inch strips
- 1 ripe tomato, chopped
- Salt and freshly ground black pepper

Directions:
1. Preparing the Ingredients
2. In a medium bowl, combine the soy sauce, 2 tablespoons of the lemon juice, and the oil. Add the portobello strips, toss to combine, and marinate for 1 hour or overnight. Drain the mushrooms and set aside.
3. To assemble wraps, place 1 tortilla on a work surface and spread with some of the mashed avocado. In the lower third of each tortilla, arrange strips of the soaked mushrooms and some of the bell pepper strips.
4. Finish and Serve
5. Sprinkle with the tomato and salt and black pepper to taste. Roll up tightly and cut in half diagonally. Repeat with the remaining Ingredients and serve.

Nutrition: Fat: 22.3 g Protein: 22.6 g Carbohydrates: 7.9 g

392. **Tamari Toasted Almonds**

Preparation Time: 2 minutes
Cooking Time: 8 minutes
Servings: ½
Ingredients:

- ½ cup raw almonds, or sunflower seeds
- 2 tablespoons tamari, or soy sauce
- 1 teaspoon toasted sesame oil

Directions:
1. Preparing the Ingredients
2. Heat a dry skillet to medium-high heat, then add the almonds, stirring frequently to keep them from burning. Once the almonds are toasted—7-8 minutes for almonds, or 34 minutes for sunflower seeds—pour the tamari and sesame oil into the hot skillet and stir to coat.
3. You can turn off the heat, and as the almonds cool the tamari mixture will stick and dry on to the nuts.

Nutrition: Calories: 89 Total fat: 8g Carbs: 3g Fiber: 2g Protein: 4g

393. **Avocado and Tempeh Bacon Wraps**

Preparation Time: 10 minutes
Cooking Time: 8 minutes
Servings: 4
Ingredients:

- 2 tablespoons extra-virgin olive oil
- 8 ounces tempeh bacon, homemade or store-bought
- 4 (10-inch) soft flour tortillas or lavish flat bread
- ¼cup vegan mayonnaise, homemade or store-bought
- 4 large lettuce leaves

- 2 ripe Hass avocados, pitted, peeled, and cut into ¼-inch slices
- 1 large ripe tomato, cut into ¼-inch slices

Directions:
1. Preparing the Ingredients
2. Cook the tempeh bacon until browned on both sides in a large skillet about 8 minutes. Remove from the heat and set aside.
3. Place 1 tortilla on a work surface. Spread with some of the mayonnaise and one-fourth of the lettuce and tomatoes.
4. Finish and Serve
5. Pit, peel, and thinly slice the avocado and place the slices on top of the tomato. Add the reserved tempeh bacon and roll up tightly. Repeat with remaining Ingredients and serve.

Nutrition: Fat: 24.3 g Protein: 11.7 g Carbohydrates: 16.7 g

394. **Kale Chips**

Preparation Time: 10 minutes
Cooking Time: 8 minutes
Servings: 4
Ingredients:

- 1 large bunch kale
- 1 tablespoon extra-virgin olive oil
- ½ teaspoon chipotle powder
- ½ teaspoon smoked paprika
- ¼ teaspoon salt

Directions:
1. Preparing the Ingredients
2. Preheat the oven to 275°F.
3. Line a large baking sheet with parchment paper. In a large bowl, stem the kale and tear it into bite-size pieces. Add the olive oil, chipotle powder, smoked paprika, and salt.
4. Toss the kale with tongs or your hands, coating each piece well.
5. Spread the kale over the parchment paper in a single layer.
6. Bake
7. Bake for 25 minutes, turning halfway through, until crisp.
8. Finish and Serve
9. Cool for 10 to 15 minutes before dividing and storing in 2 airtight containers.

Nutrition: Fat: 11 g Protein: 20.5 g Carbohydrates: 16.6 g

395. **Tempeh-Pimiento Cheese Ball**

Preparation Time: 5 minutes
Cooking Time: 30 minutes
Servings: 8
Ingredients:

- 8 ounces' tempeh, cut into ½ -inch pieces
- 1 (2-ounce) jar chopped pimientos, drained
- ¼ cup nutritional yeast
- ¼ cup vegan mayonnaise, homemade or store-bought
- 2 tablespoons soy sauce
- ¾ cup chopped pecans

Directions:

1. Preparing the Ingredients
2. In a medium saucepan of simmering water, cook the tempeh for 30 minutes. Set aside to cool. In a food processor, combine the cooled tempeh, pimientos, nutritional yeast, mayo, and soy sauce. Process until smooth.
3. Transfer the tempeh mixture to a bowl and refrigerate until firm and chilled for at least 2 hours or overnight.
4. Finish and Serve
5. In a dry skillet, toast the pecans over medium heat until lightly toasted. Set aside to cool.
6. Shape the tempeh mixture into a ball, and roll it in the pecans, pressing the nuts slightly into the tempeh mixture so they stick. Refrigerate for at least 1 hour before serving. If not using right away, cover and keep refrigerated until needed. Properly stored, it will keep for 2-3 days.

Nutrition: Fat: 9.2 g Protein: 17.6 g Carbohydrates: 4.1 g

396. **Peppers and Hummus**

Preparation Time: 15 minutes
Cooking Time: 0 minutes
Servings: 4
Ingredients:

- one 15-ounce can chickpeas, drained and rinsed
- juice of 1 lemon, or 1 tablespoon lemon juice
- ¼ cup tahini
- 3 tablespoons extra-virgin olive oil
- ½ teaspoon ground cumin
- 1 tablespoon water
- ¼ teaspoon paprika
- 1 red bell pepper, sliced
- 1 green bell pepper, sliced
- 1 orange bell pepper, sliced

Directions:
1. Preparing the Ingredients
2. In a food processor, combine chickpeas, lemon juice, tahini, 2 tablespoons of the olive oil, the cumin, and water.
3. Finish and Serve
4. Process on high speed until blended for about 30 seconds. Scoop the hummus into a bowl and drizzle with the remaining tablespoon of olive oil. Sprinkle with paprika and serve with sliced bell peppers.

Nutrition: Fat: 10 g Protein: 5.4 g Carbohydrates: 22.8 g

397. **Savory Roasted Chickpeas**

Preparation Time: 5 minutes
Cooking Time: 25 minutes
Servings: 1
Ingredients:

- 1 (14-ounce) can chickpeas, rinsed and drained, or 1½ cups cooked
- 2 tablespoons tamari, or soy sauce
- 1 tablespoon nutritional yeast
- 1 teaspoon smoked paprika, or regular paprika
- 1 teaspoon onion powder
- ½ teaspoon garlic powder

Directions:

1. Preparing the Ingredients.
2. Preheat the oven to 400°F.
3. Toss the chickpeas with all the other ingredients, and spread them out on a baking sheet.
4. Bake
5. Bake for 20-25 minutes, tossing halfway through.
6. Bake these at a lower temperature until fully dried and crispy if you want to keep them longer.
7. You can easily double the batch, and if you dry them out they will keep about a week in an airtight container.

Nutrition: Calories: 121 Total fat: 2g Carbs: 20g Fiber: 6g Protein: 8g

398. Cinnamon Spiced Popcorn
Preparation Time: 10 minutes
Cooking Time: 5 minutes
Servings: 4
Ingredients:
- 8 cups air-popped corn
- 2 teaspoons sugar
- ½ to 1 teaspoon ground cinnamon
- Butter-flavored cooking spray

Directions:
1. Preheat the oven to 350°F and line a shallow roasting pan with foil.
2. Pop the popcorn using your preferred method.
3. Spread the popcorn in the roasting pan and mix the sugar and cinnamon in a small bowl.
4. Lightly spray the popcorn with cooking spray and toss to coat evenly.
5. Sprinkle with cinnamon and toss again.
6. Bake for 5 minutes until just crisp then serve warm.

Nutrition: Calories 70 Total Fat 0.7g Saturated Fat 0.1g Total Carbs 14.7g Net Carbs 12.2g Protein 2.1g Sugar 2.2g Fiber 2.5g Sodium 1mg

399. Grilled Peaches
Preparation Time: 5 minutes
Cooking Time: 10 minutes
Servings: 6
Ingredients:
- 6 fresh peaches, ripe
- 1 tablespoon olive oil
- 6 tablespoons fat-free whipped topping

Directions:
1. Lightly grease a grill pan and preheat it over medium heat.
2. Cut the peaches in half and remove the pits.
3. Brush the cut sides with olive oil or spritz with cooking spray.
4. Place the peaches cut-side down on the grill for 4 to 5 minutes.
5. Flip the peaches and cook for another 4 to 5 minutes until tender.
6. Spoon the peaches into bowls and serve with fat-free whipped topping.

Nutrition: Calories: 100 Total Fat: 2.7g Saturated Fat: 0.3g Total Carbs: 18g Net Carbs: 15.7g, Protein:1.4g Sugar: 16g Fiber: 2.3g Sodium: 10mg

400. Peanut Butter Banana "Ice Cream"
Preparation Time: 10 minutes
Cooking Time: 0 minutes
Servings: 6
Ingredients:
- 4 medium bananas
- ½ cup whipped peanut butter
- 1 teaspoon vanilla extract

Directions:
1. Peel the bananas and slice them into coins.
2. Arrange the slices on a plate and freeze until solid.
3. Place the frozen bananas in a food processor.
4. Add the peanut butter and pulse until it is mostly smooth.
5. Scrape down the sides then add the vanilla extract.
6. Pulse until smooth then spoon into bowls to serve.

Nutrition: Calories: 165 Total Fat: 8.3 g Saturated Fat: 1.8g Total Carbs: 21.4g Net Carbs: 18g Protein: 4.9g Sugar: 11g Fiber: 3.4g Sodium: 74mg

401. Fruity Coconut Energy Balls
Preparation Time: 15 minutes
Cooking Time: 0 minutes
Servings: 18
Ingredients:
- 1 cup chopped almonds
- 1 cup dried figs
- ½ cup dried apricots, chopped
- ½ cup dried cranberries, unsweetened
- ½ teaspoon vanilla extract
- ¼ teaspoon ground cinnamon
- ½ cup shredded unsweetened coconut

Directions:
1. Place the almonds, figs, apricots, and cranberries in a food processor.
2. Pulse the mixture until finely chopped.
3. Add the vanilla extract and cinnamon then pulse to combine once more.
4. Roll the mixture into 18 small balls by hand.
5. Roll the balls in the shredded coconut and chill until firm.

Nutrition: Calories 100 Total Fat 4.9g Saturated Fat 2.1g Total Carbs 14.6g Net Carbs 11.9g Protein 1.8g Sugar 10.7g Fiber 2.7g Sodium 3mg

402. Mini Apple Oat Muffins
Preparation Time: 5 minutes
Cooking Time: 25 minutes
Servings: 24
Ingredients:
- 1 ½ cups old-fashioned oats
- 1 teaspoon baking powder
- ½ teaspoon ground cinnamon
- ¼ teaspoon baking soda
- ¼ teaspoon salt
- ½ cup unsweetened applesauce
- ¼ cup light brown sugar
- 3 tablespoons canola oil

- 3 tablespoons water
- 1 teaspoon vanilla extract
- ½ cup slivered almonds

Directions:

1. Preheat the oven to 350°F and grease a mini muffin pan.
2. Place the oats in a food processor and pulse into a fine flour.
3. Add the baking powder, cinnamon, baking soda, and salt.
4. Pulse until well combined then add the applesauce, brown sugar, canola oil, water, and vanilla then blend smooth.
5. Fold in the almonds and spoon the mixture into the muffin pan.
6. Bake for 22 to 25 minutes until a knife inserted in the center comes out clean.
7. Cool the muffins for 5 minutes then turn out onto a wire rack.

Nutrition: Calories 60 Total Fat 3.1g Saturated Fat 0.3g Total Carbs 6.5g Net Carbs 5.6g Protein 1.2g Sugar 2.1g Fiber 0.9g Sodium 38mg

403. Dark Chocolate Almond Yogurt Cups

Preparation Time: 10 minutes
Cooking Time: 0minutes
Servings: 6
Ingredients:

- 3 cups plain nonfat Greek yogurt
- ½ teaspoon almond extract
- ¼ teaspoon liquid stevia extract (more to taste)
- 2 ounces 70% dark chocolate, chopped
- ½ cup slivered almonds

Directions:

1. Whisk together the yogurt, almond extract, and liquid stevia in a medium bowl.
2. Spoon the yogurt into four dessert cups.
3. Sprinkle with chopped chocolate and slivered almonds.

Nutrition: Calories 170, Total Fat 7.7g, Saturated Fat 2.4g, Total Carbs 11.1g, Net Carbs 8.9g, Protein 14.9g, Sugar 8.1g, Fiber 2.2g, Sodium 41mg

404. Pumpkin Spice Snack Balls

Preparation Time: 15 minutes
Cooking Time: 10 minutes
Servings: 10
Ingredients:

- 1 ½ cups old-fashioned oats
- ½ cup chopped almonds
- ½ cup unsweetened shredded coconut
- ¾ cup canned pumpkin puree
- 2 tablespoons honey
- 2 teaspoons pumpkin pie spice
- ¼ teaspoon salt

Directions:

1. Preheat the oven to 300°F and line a baking sheet with parchment.

2. Combine the oats, almonds, and coconut on the baking sheet.
3. Bake for 8 to 10 minutes until browned, stirring halfway through.
4. Place the pumpkin, honey, pumpkin pie spice, and salt in a medium bowl.
5. Stir in the toasted oat mixture.
6. Shape the mixture into 20 balls by hand and place on a tray.
7. Chill until the balls are firm then serve.

Nutrition: Calories 170, Total Fat 9.8g, Saturated Fat 6g, Total Carbs 17.8g, Net Carbs 13.7g, Protein 3.8g, Sugar 5.2g, Fiber 4.1g, Sodium 64mg

405. Strawberry Lime Pudding

Preparation Time: 15 minutes
Cooking Time: 10 minutes
Servings: 4
Ingredients:

- 2 cups plus 2 tablespoons fat-free milk
- 2 teaspoons flavorless gelatin
- 10 large strawberries, sliced
- 1 tablespoon fresh lime zest
- 2 teaspoons vanilla extract
- Liquid stevia extract, to taste

Directions:

1. Whisk together 2 tablespoons milk and gelatin in a medium bowl until the gelatin dissolves completely.
2. Place the strawberries in a food processor with the lime juice and vanilla extract.
3. Blend until smooth then pour into a medium bowl.
4. Warm the remaining milk in a small saucepan over medium heat.
5. Stir in the lime zest and heat until steaming (do not boil).
6. Gently whisk the gelatin mixture into the hot milk then stir in the strawberry mixture.
7. Sweeten with liquid stevia to taste and chill until set. Serve cold.

Nutrition: Calories 75 Total Fat 0.4g, Saturated Fat 0.2g, Total Carbs 10.3, Net Carbs 9.2g, Protein 6.3g, Sugar 9.2g, Fiber 1.1g, Sodium 72mg

406. Cinnamon Toasted Almonds

Preparation Time: 5 minutes
Cooking Time: 25 minutes
Servings: 8
Ingredients:

- 2 cups whole almonds
- 1 tablespoon olive oil
- 1 teaspoon ground cinnamon
- ½ teaspoon salt

Directions:

1. Preheat the oven to 325°F and line a baking sheet with parchment.
2. Toss together the almonds, olive oil, cinnamon, and salt.
3. Spread the almonds on the baking sheet in a single layer.

4. Bake for 25 minutes, stirring several times, until toasted.

Nutrition: Calories 150, Total Fat 13.6g, Saturated Fat 1.2g Total Carbs 5.3g, Net Carbs 2.2g, Protein 5g, Sugar 1g, Fiber 3.1g, Sodium 148mg

407. Grain-Free Berry Cobbler

Preparation Time: 5 minutes
Cooking Time: 25 minutes
Servings: 10
Ingredients:

- 4 cups fresh mixed berries
- ½ cup ground flaxseed
- ¼ cup almond meal
- ¼ cup unsweetened shredded coconut
- ½ tablespoon baking powder
- 1 teaspoon ground cinnamon
- ¼ teaspoon salt
- Powdered stevia, to taste
- 6 tablespoons coconut oil

Directions:

1. Preheat the oven to 375°F and lightly grease a 10-inch cast-iron skillet.
2. Spread the berries on the bottom of the skillet.
3. Whisk together the dry ingredients in a mixing bowl.
4. Cut in the coconut oil using a fork to create a crumbled mixture.
5. Spread the crumble over the berries and bake for 25 minutes until hot and bubbling.
6. Cool the cobbler for 5 to 10 minutes before serving.

Nutrition: Calories 215 Total Fat 16.8g, Saturated Fat 10.4g, Total Carbs 13.1g, Net Carbs 6.7g, Protein 3.7g, Sugar 5.3g, Fiber 6.4g, Sodium 61mg

408. Whole-Wheat Pumpkin Muffins

Preparation Time: 15 minutes
Cooking Time: 15 minutes
Servings: 36
Ingredients:

- 1 ¾ cup whole-wheat flour
- 1 teaspoon baking powder
- 1 teaspoon baking soda
- 1 teaspoon ground cinnamon
- 1 teaspoon pumpkin pie spice
- ½ teaspoon salt
- 2 large eggs
- 1 cup canned pumpkin puree
- 1/3 cup unsweetened applesauce
- ¼ cup light brown sugar
- 1 teaspoon vanilla extract
- 1/3 cup fat-free milk
- Liquid stevia extract, to taste

Directions:

1. Preheat the oven to 350°F and grease two 24-cup mini muffin pans with cooking spray.
2. Whisk together the flour, baking powder, baking soda, cinnamon, pumpkin pie spice, and salt in a large mixing bowl.
3. In a separate bowl, whisk together the eggs, pumpkin, applesauce, brown sugar, vanilla extract, and milk.
4. Stir the wet ingredients into the dry until well combined.
5. Adjust sweetness to taste with liquid stevia extract, if desired.
6. Spoon the batter into 36 cups and bake for 12 to 15 minutes until cooked through.

Nutrition: Calories 35 Total Fat 0.5g, Saturated Fat 0.1g, Total Carbs 6.4g, Net Carbs 5.7g, Protein 1.3g, Sugar 1.6g, Fiber 0.9g, Sodium 73mg

409. Strawberry Salsa

Preparation Time: 10 minutes
Cooking Time: 5 minutes
Servings: 4
Ingredients:

- 4 tomatoes, seeded and chopped
- 1-pint strawberry, chopped
- 1 red onion, chopped
- 2 tablespoons of juice from a lime
- 1 jalapeno pepper, minced
- What you will need from the store cupboard:
- 1 tablespoon olive oil
- 2 garlic cloves, minced

Directions:

1. Bring together the strawberries, tomatoes, jalapeno, and onion in the bowl.
2. Stir in the garlic, oil, and lime juice.
3. Refrigerate. Serve with separately cooked pork or poultry.

Nutrition: Calories 19, Carbohydrates 3g, Fiber 1g, Sugar 0.2g, Cholesterol 0mg, Total Fat 1g, Protein 0g

410. Garden Wraps

Preparation Time: 20 minutes
Cooking Time: 10 minutes
Servings: 8
Ingredients:

- 1 cucumber, chopped
- 1 sweet corn
- 1 cabbage, shredded
- 1 tablespoon lettuce, minced
- 1 tomato, chopped
- What you will need from the store cupboard:
- 3 tablespoons of rice vinegar
- 2 teaspoons peanut butter
- 1/3 cup onion paste
- 1/3 cup chili sauce
- 2 teaspoons of low-sodium soy sauce

Directions:

1. Cut corn from the cob. Keep in a bowl.
2. Add the tomato, cabbage, cucumber, and onion paste.

3. Now whisk the vinegar, peanut butter, and chili sauce together.
4. Pour this over the vegetable mix. Toss for coating.
5. Let this stand for 10 minutes.
6. Take your slotted spoon and place ½ cup salad in every lettuce leaf.
7. Fold the lettuce over your filling.

Nutrition: Calories 64, Carbohydrates 13g, Fiber 2g, Sugar 1g, Cholesterol 0mg, Total Fat 1g, Protein 2g

411. **Stuffed Moroccan Mushrooms**

Preparation Time: 15 minutes
Cooking Time: 15 minutes
Servings: 12
Ingredients:

- 24 medium mushrooms
- 1/3 cup carrot, shredded
- ½ cup onion, chopped
- ½ teaspoon cumin, ground
- ¼ teaspoon coriander, ground
- What you will need from the store cupboard:
- 1 garlic clove, minced
- 1 teaspoon of canola oil
- ¾ cup vegetable broth
- ½ teaspoon salt

Directions:

1. Chop the mushroom stems finely. Keep the caps aside.
2. Sauté the chopped stems, carrot and onion in your skillet in oil until they become tender and crisp.
3. Now add the salt, garlic, coriander, and cumin.
4. Cook while stirring for a minute. Add the broth and boil.
5. Remove from heat and keep aside for 5 minutes.
6. Take a fork and fluff.
7. Place within the mushroom caps.
8. Keep on your baking sheet. Now bake for 5 minutes. The mushrooms should become tender.

Nutrition: Calories 25, Carbohydrates 5g, Fiber 1g, Sugar 1g, Cholesterol 0mg, Total Fat 0g, Protein 1g

412. **Party Shrimp**

Preparation Time: 15 minutes
Cooking Time: 10 minutes
Servings: 30
Ingredients:

- 16 oz. uncooked shrimp, peeled and deveined
- 1-1/2 teaspoons of juice from a lemon
- ½ teaspoon basil, chopped
- 1 teaspoon coriander, chopped
- ½ cup tomato
- What you will need from the store cupboard:
- 1 tablespoon of olive oil
- ½ teaspoon Italian seasoning
- ½ teaspoon paprika
- 1 sliced garlic clove
- ¼ teaspoon pepper

Directions:

1. Bring together everything except the shrimp in a dish or bowl.
2. Add the shrimp. Coat well by tossing. Set aside.
3. Drain the shrimp. Discard the marinade.
4. Keep them on a baking sheet. It should not be greased.
5. Broil each side for 4 minutes. The shrimp should become pink.

Nutrition: Calories 14 Carbohydrates 0g Fiber 0g Sugar 0g Cholesterol 18mg Total Fat 0g Protein 2g

413. **Zucchini Mini Pizzas**

Preparation Time: 20 minutes
Cooking Time: 10 minutes
Servings: 24
Ingredients:

- 1 zucchini, cut into ¼ inch slices diagonally
- ½ cup pepperoni, small slices
- 1 teaspoon basil, minced
- ½ cup onion, chopped
- 1 cup tomatoes
- What you will need from the store cupboard:
- 1/8 teaspoon pepper
- 1/8 teaspoon salt
- 3/4 cup mozzarella cheese, shredded
- 1/3 cup pizza sauce

Directions:

1. Preheat your broiler. Keep the zucchini in 1 layer on your greased baking sheet.
2. Add the onion and tomatoes. Broil each side for 1 to 2 minutes till they become tender and crisp.
3. Now sprinkle pepper and salt.
4. Top with cheese, pepperoni, and sauce.
5. Broil for a minute. The cheese should melt.
6. Sprinkle basil on top.

Nutrition: Calories 29, Carbohydrates 1g, Fiber 0g, Sugar 1g, Cholesterol 5mg, Total Fat 2g, Protein 2g

414. **Garlic-Sesame Pumpkin Seeds**

Preparation Time: 10 minutes
Cooking Time: 20 minutes
Servings: 2
Ingredients:

- 1 egg white
- 1 teaspoon onion, minced
- ½ teaspoon caraway seeds
- 2 cups pumpkin seeds
- 1 teaspoon sesame seeds
- What you will need from the store cupboard:
- 1 garlic clove, minced
- 1 tablespoon of canola oil
- ¾ teaspoon of kosher salt

Directions:

1. Preheat your oven to 350 °F.
2. Whisk together the oil and egg white in a bowl.
3. Include pumpkin seeds. Coat well by tossing.
4. Now stir in the onion, garlic, sesame seeds, caraway seeds, and salt.

5. Spread in 1 layer in your parchment-lined baking pan.
6. Bake for 15 minutes until it turns golden brown.

Nutrition: Calories 95 Carbohydrates 9g, Fiber 3g, Sugar 0g, Cholesterol 0mg, Total Fat 5g, Protein 4g

415. Roasted Eggplant Spread

Preparation Time: 10 minutes
Cooking Time: 20 minutes
Servings: 2
Ingredients:

- 1 eggplant, medium, cut into small 1 inch pieces
- 2 red peppers, cut into 1-inch pieces
- 1 red onion, cut into 1-inch pieces
- 1 tablespoon tomato
- 4 toasted baguette slices
- What you will need from the store cupboard:
- 3 garlic cloves, minced
- 3 tablespoons of olive oil
- ½ teaspoon pepper
- ½ teaspoon salt
- Cooking spray

Directions:

1. Preheat your oven to 350 °F.
2. Mix the olive oil, cloves, salt, and pepper.
3. Keep vegetables in your bowl. Now toss with the oil mix.
4. Transfer to your baking pan where you have applied cooking spray
5. Roast the vegetables till they get soft and are slightly brown.
6. Now keep in a food processor.
7. Add the tomato and pulse until it blends. The mixture must be chunky.
8. Transfer to your bowl. Serve with the baguette.

Nutrition: Calories 84 Carbohydrates 9g Fiber 3g Sugar 0.5g Cholesterol 0mg Total Fat 5g Protein 1g

416. Marinated Shrimp

Preparation Time: 10 minutes
Cooking Time: 20 minutes
Servings: 50
Ingredients:

- 30 oz. cooked shrimp, peeled and deveined
- 1 tablespoon parsley, minced
- 1/3 teaspoon dill weed
- 12 lime or lemon slices
- ½ cup red onion, sliced
- What you will need from the store cupboard:
- ½ cup lime juice
- ½ cup canola oil
- 1/8 teaspoon of hot pepper sauce
- ½ teaspoon salt

Directions:

1. Keep everything other than the shrimp in the bowl.
2. Now toss with the shrimp.
3. Set aside, stirring sometimes. Drain before you serve.

Nutrition: Calories 28 Carbohydrates 0g Fiber 0g Sugar 0g Cholesterol 26mg Total Fat 1g Protein 3g

417. Cheese and Zucchini Roulades

Preparation Time: 20 minutes
Cooking Time: 10 minutes
Servings: 24
Ingredients:

- 4 zucchini
- 2 tablespoons basil, minced
- 1 tablespoon Greek olives, chopped
- 1 teaspoon lemon zest, grated
- 1 tablespoon drained capers
- What you will need from the store cupboard:
- ¼ cup Parmesan cheese, grated
- 1 cup ricotta cheese
- 1/8 teaspoon pepper
- 1/8 teaspoon salt

Directions:

1. Mix everything except the zucchini in a bowl.
2. Slice the zucchini lengthwise into 24, 1-inch pieces.
3. Cook the zucchini pieces in batches in your greased grill rack over medium heat.
4. Grill each side for 2 to 3 minutes. They should be tender.
5. Keep the ricotta mix at the side of the zucchini slices.
6. Roll them up. Secure with toothpicks.

Nutrition: Calories 24 Carbohydrates 2g Fiber 0g Sugar 1g Cholesterol 4mg Total Fat 1g Protein 2g

418. Oatmeal Butterscotch Cookies

Preparation Time: 10 minutes
Cooking Time: 15 minutes
Serves: 4 dozen
Ingredients:

- ½ teaspoon cinnamon, ground
- 3 cups oats
- 2 eggs
- What you will need from the store cupboard:
- 1 teaspoon of baking soda
- 1-1/4 all-purpose flour
- 1 cup margarine or butter
- 1 teaspoon vanilla extract
- ½ teaspoon salt

Directions:

1. Preheat your oven to 350 °F.
2. Bring together the baking soda, flour, salt and cinnamon in a bowl.
3. Beat the eggs, vanilla extract and butter in a mixer bowl.
4. Beat in the flour mix gradually.
5. Stir in the oats.
6. Place rounded tablespoons on baking sheets. Bake for 5-6 minutes.
7. Let it cool for a couple of minutes.

Nutrition: Calories 130 Carbohydrates 16g Cholesterol 20mg Fat 7g Protein 1g Sodium 90mg

419. Party Spiced Cheese Chips

Preparation Time: 18 minutes
Cooking Time: 0 minutes
Servings: 2
Ingredients:

- 2 cups Monterrey Jack cheese, grated
- Salt to taste
- ½ tsp garlic powder
- ½ tsp cayenne pepper
- ½ tsp dried rosemary

Directions:

1. Mix grated cheese with spices. Create 2 tablespoons of cheese mixture into small mounds on a lined baking sheet. Bake for about 15 minutes at 420 F; then allow to cool to harden the chips.

Nutrition: Calories: 438 Fat 36.8g Net Carbs 1.8g Protein 27g

420. Asparagus & Chorizo Tray bake

Preparation Time: 10 minutes
Cooking Time: 20 minutes
Servings: 2
Ingredients:

- 2 tbsp olive oil
- A bunch of asparagus, ends trimmed and chopped
- 4 oz Spanish chorizo, sliced
- Salt and black pepper to taste
- ¼ cup chopped parsley

Directions:

1. Preheat your oven to 325 F and grease a baking dish with olive oil.
2. Add in the asparagus and season with salt and black pepper. Stir in the chorizo slices. Bake for 15 minutes until the chorizo is crispy. Arrange on a serving platter and serve sprinkled with parsley.

Nutrition: Calories 411 Fat: 36.5g Net Carbs: 3.2g Protein: 14.5g

421. Mortadella & Bacon Balls

Preparation Time: 25 minutes
Cooking Time: 20 minutes
Servings: 2
Ingredients:

- 4 ounces Mortadella sausage
- 4 bacon slices, cooked and crumbled
- 2 tbsp almonds, chopped
- ½ tsp Dijon mustard
- 3 ounces' cream cheese

Directions:

1. Combine the mortadella and almonds in the bowl of your food processor. Pulse until smooth. Whisk the cream cheese and mustard in another bowl. Make balls out of the mortadella mixture.
2. Make a thin cream cheese layer over. Coat with bacon, arrange on a plate and chill before serving.

Nutrition: Calories 547 Fat: 51g Net Carbs: 3.4g Protein: 21.5g

422. Speedy Italian Appetizer Balls

Preparation Time: 5 minutes
Cooking Time: 0 minutes
Servings: 2
Ingredients:

- 2 oz bresaola, chopped
- 2 oz ricotta cheese, crumbled
- 2 tbsp mayonnaise
- 6 green olives, pitted and chopped
- ½ tbsp fresh basil, finely chopped

Directions:

1. In a bowl, mix mayonnaise, bresaola and ricotta cheese. Place in fresh basil and green olives. Form balls from the mixture and refrigerate. Serve chilled.

Nutrition: Calories 175 Fat: 13.7g Net Carbs: 1.1g Protein: 11g

423. Hard-Boiled Eggs Stuffed with Ricotta Cheese

Preparation Time: 15 minutes
Cooking Time: 15 minutes
Servings: 2
Ingredients:

- 4 eggs
- 1 tbsp green tabasco
- 2 tbsp Greek yogurt
- 2 tbsp ricotta cheese
- Salt to taste

Directions:

1. Cover the eggs with salted water and bring to a boil over medium heat for 10 minutes. Place the eggs in an ice bath and let cool for 10 minutes. Peel and slice in half lengthwise. Scoop out the yolks to a bowl; mash with a fork.
2. Whisk together the tabasco, Greek yogurt, ricotta cheese, mashed yolks, and salt, in a bowl. Spoon this mixture into egg white. Arrange on a serving plate to serve.

Nutrition: Calories 173 Fat: 12.5g Net Carbs: 1.5g Protein: 13.6g

424. Delicious Egg Cups with Cheese & Spinach

Preparation Time: 10 minutes
Cooking Time: 10 minutes
Servings: 2
Ingredients:

- 4 eggs
- 1 tbsp fresh parsley, chopped
- ¼ cup cheddar cheese, shredded
- ¼ cup spinach, chopped
- Salt and black pepper to taste

Directions:

1. Grease muffin cups with cooking spray. In a bowl, whisk the eggs and add in the rest of the

ingredients. Season with salt and black pepper. Fill ¾ parts of each muffin cup with the egg mixture.

2. Bake in the oven for 15 minutes at 390 F. Serve warm!

Nutrition: Calories: 232 Fat 14.3g Net Carbs 1.5g Protein 16.2g

425. Jalapeno Turkey Tomato Bites

Preparation Time: 5 minutes
Cooking Time: 0 minutes
Servings: 2
Ingredients:

- 2 tomatoes, sliced with a 3-inch thickness
- 1 cup turkey ham, chopped
- ¼ jalapeño pepper, seeded and minced
- 1/3 tbsp Dijon mustard
- ¼ cup mayonnaise
- Salt and black pepper to taste
- 1 tbsp parsley

Directions:

1. Combine turkey ham, jalapeño pepper, mustard, mayonnaise, salt, and black pepper, in a bowl.
2. Arrange tomato slices in a single layer on a serving platter. Divide the turkey mixture between the tomato slices, garnish with parsley and serve.

Nutrition: Calories 245, Fat 15.3g, Net Carbs 6.3g, Protein 21g

426. Quail Eggs & Prosciutto Wraps

Preparation Time: 5 minutes
Cooking Time: 10 minutes
Servings: 2
Ingredients:

- 3 thin prosciutto slices
- 9 basil leaves
- 9 quail eggs

Directions:

1. Cover the quail eggs with salted water and bring to a boil over medium heat for 2-3 minutes. Place the eggs in an ice bath and let cool for 10 minutes, then peel them.
2. Cut the prosciutto slices into three strips. Place basil leaves at the end of each strip. Top with a quail egg. Wrap in prosciutto, secure with toothpicks and serve.

Nutrition: Calories 243 Fat: 21g Net Carbs: 0.5g Protein: 12.5g

427. Tomato & Cheese in Lettuce Packets

Preparation Time: 15 minutes
Cooking Time: 15 minutes
Servings: 36
Ingredients:

- ¼ pound Gruyere cheese, grated
- ¼ pound feta cheese, crumbled
- ½ tsp oregano
- 1 tomato, chopped
- ½ cup buttermilk
- ½ head lettuce

Directions:

1. In a bowl, mix feta and Gruyere cheese, oregano, tomato, and buttermilk.
2. Separate the lettuce leaves and put them on a serving platter. Divide the mixture between them, roll up, folding in the ends to secure and serve.

Nutrition: Calories 433 Fat: 32.5g Net Carbs: 6.6g Protein: 27.5g

428. Basil Mozzarella & Salami Omelet

Preparation Time: 15 minutes
Cooking Time: 15 minutes
Servings: 36
Ingredients:

- 1 tbsp butter
- 4 eggs
- 6 basils, chopped
- ½ cup mozzarella cheese
- 2 tbsp water
- 4 slices salami
- 2 tomatoes, sliced
- Salt and black pepper, to taste

Directions:

1. In a bowl, whisk the eggs with a fork. Add in the water, salt, and black pepper.
2. Melt the butter in a skillet and cook the eggs for 30 seconds. Spread the salami slices over. Arrange the sliced tomato and mozzarella over the salami. Cook for about 3 minutes. Cover the skillet and continue cooking for 3 more minutes until omelet is completely set.
3. When ready, remove the pan from heat; run a spatula around the edges of the omelet and flip it onto a warm plate, folded side down. Serve garnished with basil leaves.

Nutrition: Calories 443 Fat: 34g Net Carbs: 2.8g Protein: 29.3g

429. Pumpkin Spiced Almonds

Preparation Time: 5 minutes
Cooking Time: 25 minutes
Servings: 4
Ingredients:

- 1 tablespoon olive oil
- 1 ¼ teaspoon pumpkin pie spice
- Pinch salt
- 1 cup whole almonds, raw

Directions:

1. Preheat the oven to 300°F and line a baking sheet with parchment.
2. Whisk together the olive oil, pumpkin pie spice, and salt in a mixing bowl.
3. Toss in the almonds until evenly coated, then spread on the baking sheet.
4. Bake for 25 minutes then cool completely and store in an airtight container.

Nutrition: 170 calories 15.5g fat 5g protein 5.5g carbs 3g fiber 2.5g net carbs

430. Coco-Macadamia Fat Bombs

Preparation Time: 5 minutes
Cooking Time: 0 minutes
Servings: 16
Ingredients:

- 1 cup coconut oil
- 1 cup smooth almond butter
- ½ cup unsweetened cocoa powder
- ¼ cup coconut flour
- Liquid stevia extract, to taste
- 16 whole macadamia nuts, raw

Directions:

1. Melt the coconut oil and cashew butter together in a small saucepan.
2. Whisk in the cocoa powder, coconut flour, and liquid stevia to taste.
3. Remove from heat and let cool until it hardens slightly.
4. Divide the mixture into 16 even pieces.
5. Roll each piece into a ball around a macadamia nut and chill until ready to eat.

Nutrition: 255 calories 25.5g fat 3.5g protein 7g carbs 3g fiber 4g net carbs

431. Tzatziki Dip with Cauliflower

Preparation Time: 10 minutes
Cooking Time: 0 minutes
Servings: 6
Ingredients:

- ½ (8-ounce) package cream cheese, softened
- 1 cup sour cream
- 1 tablespoon ranch seasoning
- 1 English cucumber, diced
- 2 tablespoons chopped chives
- 2 cups cauliflower florets

Directions:

1. Beat the cream cheese with an electric mixer until creamy.
2. Add the sour cream and ranch seasoning, then beat until smooth.
3. Fold in the cucumbers and chives, then chill before serving with cauliflower florets for dipping.

Nutrition: 125 calories 10.5g fat 3g protein 5.5g carbs 1g fiber 4.5g net carbs

432. Curry-Roasted Macadamia Nuts

Preparation Time: 5 minutes
Cooking Time: 25 minutes
Servings: 8
Ingredients:

- 1 ½ tablespoons olive oil
- 1 tablespoon curry powder
- ½ teaspoon salt
- 2 cups macadamia nuts, raw

Directions:

1. Preheat the oven to 300°F and line a baking sheet with parchment.
2. Whisk together the olive oil, curry powder, and salt in a mixing bowl.
3. Toss in the macadamia nuts to coat, then spread on the baking sheet.
4. Bake for 25 minutes until toasted, then cool to room temperature.

Nutrition: 265 calories 28g fat 3g protein 5g carbs 3g fiber 2g net carbs

433. Sesame Almond Fat Bombs

Preparation Time: 5 minutes
Cooking Time: 0 minutes
Servings: 16
Ingredients:

- 1 cup coconut oil
- 1 cup smooth almond butter
- ½ cup unsweetened cocoa powder
- ¼ cup almond flour
- Liquid stevia extract, to taste
- ½ cup toasted sesame seeds

Directions:

1. Combine the coconut oil and almond butter in a small saucepan.
2. Cook over low heat until melted, then whisk in the cocoa powder, almond flour, and liquid stevia.
3. Remove from heat and let cool until it hardens slightly.
4. Divide the mixture into 16 even pieces and roll into balls.
5. Roll the balls in the toasted sesame seeds and chill until ready to eat.

Nutrition: 260 calories 26g fat 4g protein 6g carbs 2g fiber 4g net carbs

434. Coconut Chia Pudding

Preparation Time: 5 minutes
Cooking Time: 0 minutes
Servings: 6
Ingredients:

- 2 ¼ cup canned coconut milk
- 1 teaspoon vanilla extract
- Pinch salt
- ½ cup chia seeds

Directions:

1. Combine the coconut milk, vanilla, and salt in a bowl.
2. Stir well and sweeten with stevia to taste.
3. Whisk in the chia seeds and chill overnight.
4. Spoon into bowls and serve with chopped nuts or fruit.

Nutrition: 300 calories 27.5g fat 6g protein 14.5g carbs 10g fiber 4.5g net carbs

435. Chocolate Almond Butter Brownies

Preparation Time: 15 minutes
Cooking Time: 30minutes
Servings: 16
Ingredients:

- 1 cup almond flour

- ¾ cup unsweetened cocoa powder
- ½ cup shredded unsweetened coconut
- ½ teaspoon baking soda
- 1 cup coconut oil
- ½ cup canned coconut milk
- 2 large eggs
- 1 ½ teaspoons liquid stevia extract
- ¼ cup almond butter

Directions:
1. Preheat the oven to 350°F and line a square pan with foil.
2. Whisk together the almond flour, cocoa powder, coconut, and baking soda in a mixing bowl.
3. In another bowl, beat together the coconut oil, coconut milk, eggs, and liquid stevia.
4. Stir the wet ingredients into the dry until just combined, then spread in the pan.
5. Melt the almond butter in the microwave until creamy.
6. Drizzle over the chocolate batter, then swirl gently with a knife.
7. Bake for 25 to 30 minutes until the center is set then cool completely, then cut into 16 equal pieces.

Nutrition: 200 calories 21g fat 3g protein 4.5g carbs 2.5g fiber 2g net carbs

436. **Blueberry Popovers**

Preparation Time: 20 minutes
Cooking Time: 30 minutes
Servings: 8
Ingredients:
- 1 cup all-purpose flour
- pinch salt
- 2 eggs
- 1 cup 1 percent milk
- 1/2 cup blueberries
- 1 tbsp icing sugar to dust
- Berry Salad
- 1 cup raspberries
- 1 cup blueberries
- 1 cup strawberries hulled and thickly sliced

Directions:
1. Preheat the oven to 425°F (220°C). Using nonstick cooking spray, grease 8 cups of a 12-cup muffin pan (each cup should measure about 6 cm across the top and be about 3 cm deep).
2. Sift the flour and salt into a mixing bowl, add the sugar, and make a well in the center. Break the eggs into the well, add the milk and beat together with a fork.
3. Using a wire whisk, gradually work the flour into the liquid to make a smooth batter.
4. Divide the batter evenly among the prepared muffin cups: they should be about two-thirds full. With a spoon, drop a few blueberries into the batter in each cup, dividing them equally. Half-fill the 4 empty cups with water.

5. Bake in the center of the oven for 25 to 30 minutes or until the popovers are golden-brown, risen and crisp around the edges.
6. Meanwhile, to make the Berry salad, purée two-thirds of the raspberries by pressing them through a nylon sieve into a bowl. Add the remaining raspberries to the bowl, together with the blueberries and strawberries. Sift the icing sugar over the fruit and fold gently to mix everything together.
7. Remove the popovers with a round-bladed knife, and dust with the icing sugar. Serve the blueberry popovers hot, with the berry salad.

Nutrition: 100 calories 23g fat 3g protein 4.5g carbs 2.5g fiber 2g net carbs

437. **Nutty wild Rice Salad**

Preparation Time: 20 minutes
Cooking Time: 40 minutes
Servings: 8
Ingredients:
- 2/3 cup uncooked wild rice
- cans (14 ounces) sauerkraut rinsed and well drained
- 1 medium apple peeled and chopped
- 3/4 cup celery chopped
- 3/4 cup carrot shredded (about 1 large carrot)
- 1/2 cup red onion finely chopped
- Dressing
- 1/2 cup sugar
- 1/3 cup cider vinegar
- 1 tbsp canola oil
- 1/4 tsp salt
- 1/4 tsp pepper
- 1 tbsp fresh parsley minced
- 1 tbsp fresh tarragon minced (or 1 tsp dried tarragon)
- 3/4 cup walnuts chopped, toasted

Directions:
1. 1 Cook wild rice according to package directions. Cool completely.
2. In a large bowl, combine sauerkraut, apple, celery, carrot, onion and cooled rice. In a small bowl, whisk the first five dressing ingredients until sugar is dissolved; stir in herbs. Add to sauerkraut mixture; toss to combine.
3. Refrigerate, covered, at least 4 hours to allow flavours to blend. Stir in walnuts just before serving.
4. Tip: To toast nuts, bake in a shallow pan in a 350° oven for 5-10 minutes or cook in a skillet over low heat until lightly browned, stirring occasionally.

Nutrition: 300 calories 27.5g fat 6g protein 14.5g carbs 10g fiber 4.5g net carbs

438. **Apricot and Pecan Muffies**

Preparation Time: 25 minutes
Cooking Time: 20 minutes
Servings: 12
Ingredients:
- 1/4 cups almond flour
- 1 tbsp wheat bran

- 1 tbsp baking powder
- 1 tsp ground cinnamon
- 1/2 tsp lemon zest grated
- 1/4 tsp salt
- eggs large
- tbsp unsalted butter light, melted and cooled
- 1 cup skim milk
- apricots peeled, pitted and coarsely chopped
- 1/4 cup chopped pecans

Directions:

1. 1 Preheat the oven to 375F (190C). Lightly coat a 12-cup muffin pan with cooking spray or line with paper baking cups.
2. In a large bowl, mix the flour, sugar, wheat bran, baking powder, cinnamon, lemon zest and salt. Make a well in the centre of the dry ingredients and set aside.
3. In a large measuring cup, whisk the eggs until frothy and light yellow. Beat in the butter, then the milk, until well blended. Pour this mixture into the well in the centre of the flour mixture. Stir just until the dry ingredients are moistened. The batter will be slightly lumpy. Do not overmix the batter or the muffins will be tough. With a rubber spatula, gently fold in the apricots and pecans.
4. Spoon the batter into the prepared muffin pan, filling the cups 3/4 full. Bake the muffins until they are peaked and golden brown, about 20 minutes. The muffins are done when a wooden toothpick inserted in the centre comes out almost clean, with a few moist crumbs clinging to it. Let the muffins cool in the pan for 3 minutes before removing them. These muffins are best when served piping hot or within a few hours of baking.

Nutrition: 255 calories 25.5g fat 3.5g protein 7g carbs 3g fiber 4g net carbs

DESSERT RECIPES

439. Pumpkin & Banana Ice Cream

Preparation Time: 5 minutes
Cooking Time: 10 minutes
Servings: 4
Ingredients:

- 15 oz. pumpkin puree
- 4 bananas, sliced and frozen
- 1 teaspoon pumpkin pie spice
- Chopped pecans

Directions:

1. Add pumpkin puree, bananas and pumpkin pie spice in a food processor.
2. Pulse until smooth.
3. Chill in the refrigerator.
4. Garnish with pecans.

Nutrition: Calories 71 Total Fat 0.4 g Total Carbohydrate 18 g Protein 1.2 g

440. Brûléed Oranges

Preparation Time: 5 minutes
Cooking Time: 10 minutes
Servings: 4
Ingredients:

- 4 oranges, sliced into segments
- 1 teaspoon ground cardamom
- 6 teaspoons brown sugar
- 1 cup nonfat Greek yogurt

Directions:

1. Preheat your broiler.
2. Arrange orange slices in a baking pan.
3. In a bowl, mix the cardamom and sugar.
4. Sprinkle mixture on top of the oranges. Broil for 5 minutes.
5. Serve oranges with yogurt.

Nutrition: Calories 168 Total Fat 4.2 g Total Carbohydrate 26.9 g Protein 6.8 g

441. Frozen Lemon & Blueberry

Preparation Time: 5 minutes
Cooking Time: 10 minutes
Servings: 4
Ingredients:

- 6 cup fresh blueberries
- 8 sprigs fresh thyme
- ¾ cup light brown sugar
- 1 teaspoon lemon zest
- ¼ cup lemon juice
- 2 cups water

Directions:

1. Add blueberries, thyme and sugar in a pan over medium heat.
2. Cook for 6 to 8 minutes.
3. Transfer mixture to a blender.
4. Remove thyme sprigs.
5. Stir in the remaining ingredients.
6. Pulse until smooth.
7. Strain mixture and freeze for 1 hour.

Nutrition: Calories 78 Total Fat 0 g Total Carbohydrate 20 g Protein 3 g

442. Peanut Butter Choco Chip Cookies

Preparation Time: 5 minutes
Cooking Time: 10 minutes
Servings: 4
Ingredients:

- 1 egg
- ½ cup light brown sugar
- 1 cup natural unsweetened peanut butter
- Pinch salt
- ¼ cup dark chocolate chips

Directions:

1. Preheat your oven to 375 degrees F.
2. Mix egg, sugar, peanut butter, salt and chocolate chips in a bowl.
3. Form into cookies and place in a baking pan.
4. Bake the cookie for 10 minutes.
5. Let cool before serving.

Nutrition: Calories 159 Total Fat 10 g Total Carbohydrate 12 g Protein 4.3 g

443. Watermelon Sherbet

Preparation Time: 5 minutes
Cooking Time: 3 minutes
Servings: 4
Ingredients:

- 6 cups watermelon, sliced into cubes
- 14 oz. almond milk
- 1 tablespoon honey
- ¼ cup lime juice
- Salt to taste

Directions:

1. Freeze watermelon for 4 hours.
2. Add frozen watermelon and other ingredients in a blender.
3. Blend until smooth.
4. Transfer to a container with seal.
5. Seal and freeze for 4 hours.

Nutrition: Calories 132 Total Fat 3 g Total Carbohydrate 24.5 g Protein 3.1 g

444. Strawberry & Mango Ice Cream

Preparation Time: 5 minutes
Cooking Time: 10 minutes
Servings: 4
Ingredients:

- 8 oz. strawberries, sliced
- 12 oz. mango, sliced into cubes
- 1 tablespoon lime juice

Directions:

1. Add all ingredients in a food processor.
2. Pulse for 2 minutes.
3. Chill before serving.

Nutrition: Calories 70 Total Fat 0.5 g Total Carbohydrate 17.4 g Protein 1.1 g

445. Sparkling Fruit Drink: Diabetic

Preparation Time: 5 minutes
Cooking Time: 10 minutes
Servings: 4
Ingredients:

- 8 oz. unsweetened grape juice
- 8 oz. unsweetened apple juice
- 8 oz. unsweetened orange juice
- 1 qt. homemade ginger ale
- Ice

Directions:

1. Makes 7 servings. Mix first 4 ingredients together in a pitcher. Add ice cubes and 9 ounces of the beverage to each glass. Serve immediately.

Nutrition: Calories 60 Protein 1.1 g

446. Tiramisu Shots

Preparation Time: 5 minutes
Cooking Time: 10 minutes
Servings: 4
Ingredients:

- 1 pack silken tofu
- 1 oz. dark chocolate, finely chopped
- ¼ cup sugar substitute
- 1 teaspoon lemon juice
- ¼ cup brewed espresso
- Pinch salt
- 24 slices angel food cake
- Cocoa powder (unsweetened)

Directions:

1. Add tofu, chocolate, sugar substitute, lemon juice, espresso and salt in a food processor.
2. Pulse until smooth.
3. Add angel food cake pieces into shot glasses.
4. Drizzle with the cocoa powder.
5. Pour the tofu mixture on top.
6. Top with the remaining angel food cake pieces.
7. Chill for 30 minutes and serve.

Nutrition: Calories 75 Total Fat 1.8 g Total Carbohydrate 12 g Protein 2.9 g

447. Ice Cream Brownie Cake

Preparation Time: 5 minutes
Cooking Time: 10 minutes
Servings: 4
Ingredients:

- Cooking spray
- 12 oz. no-sugar brownie mix
- ¼ cup oil
- 2 egg whites
- 3 tablespoons water
- 2 cups sugar-free ice cream

Directions:

1. Preheat your oven to 325 degrees F.
2. Spray your baking pan with oil.

3. Mix brownie mix, oil, egg whites and water in a bowl.
4. Pour into the baking pan.
5. Bake for 25 minutes.
6. Let cool.
7. Freeze brownie for 2 hours.
8. Spread ice cream over the brownie.
9. Freeze for 8 hours.

Nutrition: Calories 198 Total Fat 10 g Total Carbohydrate 33 g Protein 3 g

448. Peanut Butter Cups

Preparation Time: 5 minutes
Cooking Time: 10 minutes
Servings: 4
Ingredients:

- 1 packet plain gelatin
- ¼ cup sugar substitute
- 2 cups nonfat cream
- ½ teaspoon vanilla
- ¼ cup low-fat peanut butter
- 2 tablespoons unsalted peanuts, chopped

Directions:

1. Mix gelatin, sugar substitute and cream in a pan.
2. Let sit for 5 minutes.
3. Place over medium heat and cook until gelatin has been dissolved.
4. Stir in vanilla and peanut butter.
5. Pour into custard cups. Chill for 3 hours.
6. Top with the peanuts and serve.

Nutrition: Calories 171 Total Fat 5.6 g Total Carbohydrate 21 g Protein 6.8 g

449. Fruit Pizza

Preparation Time: 5 minutes
Cooking Time: 10 minutes
Servings: 4
Ingredients:

- 1 teaspoon maple syrup
- ¼ teaspoon vanilla extract
- ½ cup coconut milk yogurt
- 2 round slices watermelon
- ½ cup blackberries, sliced
- ½ cup strawberries, sliced
- 2 tablespoons coconut flakes (unsweetened)

Directions:

1. Mix maple syrup, vanilla and yogurt in a bowl.
2. Spread the mixture on top of the watermelon slice.
3. Top with the berries and coconut flakes.

Nutrition: Calories 70 Total Carbohydrate 14.6 g Protein 1.2 g

450. Choco Peppermint Cake

Preparation Time: 5 minutes
Cooking Time: 10 minutes
Servings: 4
Ingredients:

- Cooking spray
- ⅓ cup oil
- 15 oz. package chocolate cake mix

- 3 eggs, beaten
- 1 cup water
- ¼ teaspoon peppermint extract

Directions:
1. Spray slow cooker with oil.
2. Mix all the ingredients in a bowl.
3. Use an electric mixer on medium speed setting to mix ingredients for 2 minutes.
4. Pour mixture into the slow cooker.
5. Cover the pot and cook on low for 3 hours.
6. Let cool before slicing and serving.

Nutrition: Calories 185 Total Fat 7.4 g Total Carbohydrate 27 g Protein 3.8 g

451. Roasted Mango

Preparation Time: 5 minutes
Cooking Time: 10 minutes
Servings: 4
Ingredients:

- 2 mangoes, sliced
- 2 teaspoons crystallized ginger, chopped
- 2 teaspoons orange zest
- 2 tablespoons coconut flakes (unsweetened)

Directions:
1. Preheat your oven to 350 degrees F.
2. Add mango slices in custard cups.
3. Top with the ginger, orange zest and coconut flakes.
4. Bake in the oven for 10 minutes.

Nutrition: Calories 89 Total Fat 1.5 g Total Carbohydrate 20 g Protein 0.8 g

452. Roasted Plums

Preparation Time: 5 minutes
Cooking Time: 10 minutes
Servings: 4
Ingredients:

- Cooking spray
- 6 plums, sliced
- ½ cup pineapple juice (unsweetened)
- 1 tablespoon brown sugar
- 2 tablespoons brown sugar
- ¼ teaspoon ground cardamom
- ½ teaspoon ground cinnamon
- ⅛ teaspoon ground cumin

Directions:
1. Combine all the ingredients in a baking pan.
2. Roast in the oven at 450 degrees F for 20 minutes.

Nutrition: Calories 102 Total Fat 2.7 g Total Carbohydrate 18.7 g Protein 2 g

453. Figs with Honey & Yogurt

Preparation Time: 5 minutes
Cooking Time: 10 minutes
Servings: 4
Ingredients:

- ½ teaspoon vanilla
- 8 oz. nonfat yogurt
- 2 figs, sliced
- 1 tablespoon walnuts, chopped and toasted

- 2 teaspoons honey

Directions:
1. Stir vanilla into yogurt.
2. Mix well.
3. Top with the figs and sprinkle with walnuts.
4. Drizzle with honey and serve.

Nutrition: Calories 157 Total Fat 4 g Total Carbohydrate 24 g Protein 7 g

454. Strawberry Shake

Preparation Time: 10 minutes
Cooking time: 10 minutes
Servings: 2
Ingredients:

- 1½ cups fresh strawberries, hulled
- 1 large frozen banana, peeled
- 2 scoops unsweetened vegan vanilla protein powder
- 2 tablespoons hemp seeds
- 2 cups unsweetened hemp milk

Directions:
1. In a high-speed blender, place all the ingredients and pulse until creamy.
2. Pour into two glasses and serve immediately.

Nutrition: Calories 325 Total Fat 13 g Saturated Fat 0.8 g Cholesterol 0 mg Sodium 391 mg Total Carbs 23.3 g Fiber 3.9 g Sugar 12.5 g Protein 31.2 g

455. Chocolatey Banana Shake

Preparation Time: 10 minutes
Cooking time: 10 minutes
Servings: 2
Ingredients:

- 2 medium frozen bananas, peeled
- 4 dates, pitted
- 4 tablespoons peanut butter
- 4 tablespoons rolled oats
- 2 tablespoons cacao powder
- 2 tablespoons chia seeds
- 2 cups unsweetened soymilk

Directions:
1. Place all the ingredients in a high-speed blender and pulse until creamy.
2. Pour into two glasses and serve immediately.

Nutrition: Calories 583 Total Fat 25.2 g Saturated Fat 4.8 g Cholesterol 0 mg Sodium 200 mg Total Carbs 75 g Fiber 15.3 g Sugar 37.8 g Protein 23.1 g

456. Fruity Tofu Smoothie

Preparation Time: 10 minutes
Cooking time: 10 minutes
Servings: 2
Ingredients:

- 12 ounces' silken tofu, pressed and drained
- 2 medium bananas, peeled
- 1½ cups fresh blueberries
- 1 tablespoon maple syrup
- 1½ cups unsweetened soymilk
- ¼ cup ice cubes

Directions:

1. Place all the ingredients in a high-speed blender and pulse until creamy.
2. Pour into two glasses and serve immediately.

Nutrition: Calories 398 Total Fat 8.6 g Saturated Fat 1.2 g Cholesterol 0 mg Sodium 58 mg Total Carbs 65 g Fiber 7 g Sugar 50.7 g Protein 19.9 g

457. Green Fruity Smoothie

Preparation Time: 10 minutes
Cooking time: 10 minutes
Servings: 2
Ingredients:

- 1 cup frozen mango, peeled, pitted, and chopped
- 1 large frozen banana, peeled
- 2 cups fresh baby spinach
- 1 scoop unsweetened vegan vanilla protein powder
- ¼ cup pumpkin seeds
- 2 tablespoons hemp hearts
- 1½ cups unsweetened almond milk

Directions:

1. In a high-speed blender, place all the ingredients and pulse until creamy.
2. Pour into two glasses and serve immediately.

Nutrition: Calories 355 Total Fat 16.1 g Saturated Fat 2.4 g Cholesterol 0 mg Sodium 295 mg Total Carbs 34.6 g Fiber 6.2 g Sugar 19.9 g Protein 23.4 g

458. Protein Latte

Preparation Time: 10 minutes
Cooking time: 10 minutes
Servings: 2
Ingredients:

- 2 cups hot brewed coffee
- 1¼ cups coconut milk
- 2 teaspoons coconut oil
- 2 scoops unsweetened vegan vanilla protein powder

Directions:

1. Place all the ingredients in a high-speed blender and pulse until creamy.
2. Pour into two serving mugs and serve immediately.

Nutrition: Calories 503 Total Fat 41.4 g Saturated Fat 35.6 g Cholesterol 0 mg Sodium 291 mg Total Carbs 8.3 g Fiber 3.3 g Sugar 5 g Protein 29.1 g

459. Chocolatey Bean Mousse

Preparation Time: 10 minutes
Cooking time: 10 minutes
Servings: 3
Ingredients:

- ½ cup unsweetened almond milk
- 1 cup cooked black beans
- 4 Medjool dates, pitted and chopped
- ½ cup walnuts, chopped
- 2 tablespoons cacao powder
- 1 teaspoon vanilla extract
- 3 tablespoons fresh blueberries
- 1 teaspoon fresh mint leaves

Directions:

1. In a food processor, add all ingredients and pulse until smooth and creamy.

2. Transfer the mousse into serving bowls and refrigerate to chill before serving.
3. Garnish with blueberries and mint leaves and serve.

Nutrition: Calories 465 Total Fat 14.5 g Saturated Fat 1.4 g Cholesterol 0 mg Sodium 34 mg Total Carbs 69.9 g Fiber 15 g Sugar 23.3 g Protein 21.1 g

460. Tofu & Strawberry Mousse

Preparation Time: 10 minutes
Cooking time: 10 minutes
Servings: 4
Ingredients:

- 2 cups fresh strawberries, hulled and sliced
- 2 cups firm tofu, pressed and drained
- 3 tablespoons maple syrup
- 4 tablespoons walnuts, chopped

Directions:

1. In a blender, add the strawberries and pulse until just pureed.
2. Add the tofu and maple syrup and pulse until smooth.
3. Transfer the mousse into serving bowls and refrigerate to chill before serving.
4. Garnish with walnuts and serve.

Nutrition: Calories 199 Total Fat 10.1 g Saturated Fat 1.4 g Cholesterol 0 mg Sodium 17 mg Total Carbs 18.5 g Fiber 3.1 g Sugar 13.3 g Protein 12.7 g

461. Tofu & Chia Seed Pudding

Preparation Time: 15 minutes
Cooking Time: 15 minutes
Servings: 4
Ingredients:

- 1-pound silken tofu, pressed and drained
- ¼ cup banana, peeled
- 3 tablespoons cacao powder
- 1 teaspoon vanilla extract
- 3 tablespoons chia seeds
- ¼ cup walnuts, chopped
- ¼ cup black raisins

Directions:

1. In a food processor, add tofu, banana, cocoa powder, and vanilla, and pulse till smooth and creamy.
2. Transfer into a large serving bowl and stir in chia seeds till well mixed.
3. Now, place the pudding in serving bowls evenly.
4. With plastic wraps, cover the bowls. Refrigerate to chill before serving.
5. Garnish with raspberries and serve.

Nutrition: Calories 188 Total Fat 10.4 g Saturated Fat 1.4 g Cholesterol 0 mg Sodium 42 mg Total Carbs 17.1 g Fiber 4.2 g Sugar 8.2 g Protein 12 g

462. Banana Brownies

Preparation Time: 15 minutes
Cooking time: 20 minutes
Servings: 8
Ingredients:

- 6 bananas
- 2 scoops unsweetened vegan vanilla protein powder

- 1 cup creamy peanut butter
- ½ cup cacao powder

Directions:
1. Preheat the oven the 350ºF. Line a square baking dish with greased parchment paper.
2. In a food processor, add all the ingredients and pulse until smooth.
3. Transfer the mixture into the baking dish evenly and with the back of a spatula, smooth the top surface.
4. Bake for about 18–20 minutes.
5. Remove from oven and place onto a wire rack to cool completely.
6. With a sharp knife, cut into equal-sized brownies and serve.

Nutrition: Calories 310 Total Fat 17.8 g Saturated Fat 4.2 g Cholesterol 0 mg Sodium 215 mg Total Carbs 29.1 g Fiber 5.7 g Sugar 13.7 g Protein 16.4 g

463. Brown Rice Pudding

Preparation Time: 15 minutes
Cooking time: 1¼ hours
Servings: 2
Ingredients:

- ½ cup brown basmati rice, soaked for 15 minutes and drained
- 1½ cups water
- 2½ cups unsweetened almond milk
- 4 tablespoons cashews
- 2–3 tablespoons maple syrup
- 1/8 teaspoon ground cardamom
- Pinch of salt
- 3 tablespoons golden raisins
- 2 tablespoons cashews
- 2 tablespoons almonds

Directions:
1. In a pan, add the rice and water over medium-high heat and bring to a boil.
2. Lower the heat to medium and cook for about 30 minutes.
3. Meanwhile, in a blender, add the almond milk and cashews and pulse until smooth.
4. In the pan of rice, slowly add the milk mixture stirring continuously.
5. Sir in the maple syrup, cardamom, and salt, and cook for about 15–20 minutes, stirring occasionally.
6. Stir in the raisins and cook for about 15–20 minutes, stirring occasionally.
7. Remove from the heat and set aside to cool slightly.
8. Serve warm with the garnishing of banana slices and pistachios.

Nutrition: Calories 498 Total Fat 20.7 g Saturated Fat 3.2 g Cholesterol 0 mg Sodium 317 mg Total Carbs 72.7 g Fiber 4.9 g Sugar 21.5 g Protein 10.5 g

464. Chocó Muffins

Preparation Time: 10 minutes
Cooking Time: 20 minutes
Servings: 12
Ingredients:

- 4 eggs
- 1 tsp vanilla
- ¼ cup butter
- 1 tsp baking powder
- ¼ cup heavy cream
- ¼ cup erythritol
- 1 oz unsweetened chocolate chips
- 1 oz unsweetened chocolate, chopped
- ¼ cup unsweetened cocoa powder
- ½ cup almond flour
- Pinch of salt

Directions:
1. Spray a muffin tray with cooking spray and set aside.
2. In a bowl, mix together almond flour, baking powder, sweetener, cocoa powder, and salt.
3. In a separate bowl, beat together butter and heavy cream.
4. Add vanilla and eggs and beat until well combined.
5. Add almond flour mixture to the egg mixture and mix well to combine.
6. Add chopped chocolate and chocolate chips and fold well.
7. Pour batter in a muffin tray and bake at 350 F/ 180 C for 20 minutes.
8. Serve and enjoy.

Nutrition: Calories 123 Fat 11.3 g Carbohydrates 3.7 g Sugar 0.4 g Protein 3.9 g Cholesterol 68 mg

465. Chia Strawberry Pudding

Preparation Time: 10 minutes
Cooking Time: 10 minutes
Servings: 4
Ingredients:

- 1 tsp unsweetened cocoa powder
- 5 tbsp chia seeds
- 2 tbsp xylitol
- 1 1/2 tsp vanilla
- 1 ½ cups strawberries, chopped
- 1 cup unsweetened coconut milk
- Pinch of salt

Directions:
1. In a saucepan, combine together strawberries, ½ cup water, xylitol, vanilla, and salt and simmer over medium heat for 5-10 minutes.
2. Mash strawberries with a fork.
3. Add coconut milk and stir to combine.
4. Add chia seeds and mix well and let it sit for 5 minutes.
5. Pour pudding mixture in serving glasses.
6. Sprinkle cocoa powder on top of chia pudding.
7. Place in refrigerator for 1 hour.
8. Serve chilled and enjoy.

Nutrition: Calories 211 Fat 17.4 g Carbohydrates 11 g Sugar 4.9 g Protein 3.8 g Cholesterol 0 mg

466. Cinnamon Protein Bars

Preparation Time: 10 minutes
Cooking Time: 10 minutes

Servings: 8

Ingredients:

- 2 scoops vanilla protein powder
- 1/4 cup coconut oil, melted
- 1 cup almond butter
- 1/4 tsp cinnamon
- 12 drops liquid stevia
- Pinch of salt

Directions:

1. In a bowl, mix together all ingredients until well combined.
2. Transfer bar mixture into a baking dish and press down evenly.
3. Place in refrigerator until firm.
4. Slice and serve.

Nutrition: Calories 99 Fat 8 g Carbohydrates 0.6 g Sugar 0.2 g Protein 7.2 g Cholesterol 0 mg

467. Chocolate Cake

Preparation Time: 10 minutes

Cooking Time: 30 minutes

Servings: 12

Ingredients:

- 5 large eggs
- 1 1/2 cup erythritol
- 10 oz unsweetened chocolate, melted
- 1/2 cup almond flour
- 10 oz butter, melted
- Pinch of salt

Directions:

1. Preheat the oven to 350 F/ 180 C.
2. Grease spring-form cake pan with butter and set aside.
3. In a large bowl, beat eggs until foamy.
4. Add erythritol and stir well.
5. Add melted butter, chocolate, almond flour, and salt and stir to combine.
6. Pour batter in the cake pan and bake in preheated oven for 30 minutes.
7. Remove cake from oven and allow to cool completely.
8. Slice and serve.

Nutrition: Calories 344 Fat 35 g Carbohydrates 8 g Sugar 0.6 g Protein 6.9 g Cholesterol 128 mg

468. Raspberry Almond Tart

Preparation Time: 10 minutes

Cooking Time: 23 minutes

Servings: 4

Ingredients:

- 5 egg whites
- 1 tsp vanilla
- 1 1/2 cups raspberries
- 1 lemon zest, grated
- 1 cup almond flour
- 1/2 cup Swerve
- 1/2 cup butter, melted
- 1 tsp baking powder

Directions:

1. Preheat the oven to 375 F/ 190 C.
2. Grease tart tin with cooking spray and set aside.
3. In a large bowl, whisk egg whites until foamy.
4. Add sweetener, baking powder, vanilla, lemon zest, and almond flour and mix until well combined.
5. Add melted butter and stir well.
6. Pour batter in tart tin and top with raspberries.
7. Bake in preheated oven for 20-23 minutes.
8. Serve and enjoy.

Nutrition: Calories 378 Fat 8 g Carbohydrates 14 g Sugar 4 g Protein 11 g Cholesterol 0 mg

469. Vanilla Ice Cream

Preparation Time: 10 minutes

Cooking Time: 30 minutes

Servings: 8

Ingredients:

- 1 egg yolk
- 3/4 cup erythritol
- 2 cups heavy whipping cream
- 1 tsp vanilla
- 3 tsp cinnamon
- Pinch of salt

Directions:

1. Add all ingredients to the mixing bowl and blend until well combined.
2. Pour ice cream mixture into the ice cream maker and churn ice cream according to the machine instructions.
3. Serve and enjoy.

Nutrition: Calories 114 Fat 11.7 g Carbohydrates 1.7 g Sugar 0.1 g Protein 1 g Cholesterol 67 mg

470. Fresh Berry Yogurt

Preparation Time: 10 minutes

Cooking Time: 10 minutes

Servings: 6

Ingredients:

- 1 tsp vanilla
- 1 cup coconut cream
- 1 cup mixed berries
- 2 tbsp erythritol
- 1/2 lemon juice

Directions:

1. In a bowl, mix together coconut cream, sweetener, lemon juice, and vanilla and place in the refrigerator for 30 minutes.
2. Add berries and frozen coconut cream mixture into the blender and blend until smooth.
3. Transfer blended mixture in container and place in the refrigerator for 1-2 hours.
4. Serve and enjoy.

Nutrition: Calories 100 Fat 9 g Carbohydrates 5 g Sugar 3.2 g Protein 1 g Cholesterol 0 mg

471. Cheese Berry Fat Bomb

Preparation Time: 5 minutes

Cooking Time: 5 minutes

Servings: 12

Ingredients:

- 1 cup fresh berries, wash

- 1/2 cup coconut oil
- 1 1/2 cup cream cheese, softened
- 1 tbsp vanilla
- 2 tbsp swerve

Directions:
1. Add all ingredients to the blender and blend until smooth and combined.
2. Spoon mixture into small candy molds and refrigerate until set.
3. Serve and enjoy.

Nutrition: Calories 175 Fat 17 g Carbohydrates 2 g Sugar 1 g Protein 2.1 g Cholesterol 29 mg

472. Chocó Cookies

Preparation Time: 10 minutes
Cooking Time: 10 minutes
Servings: 14
Ingredients:
- 1 egg
- 1/2 cup erythritol
- 1/4 cup unsweetened cocoa powder
- 1 cup almond butter
- 3 tbsp unsweetened almond milk
- 1/4 cup unsweetened chocolate chips

Directions:
1. Preheat the oven to 350 F/ 180 C.
2. Line baking tray with parchment paper and set aside.
3. In a bowl, mix together almond butter, egg, sweetener, almond milk, and cocoa powder until well combined.
4. Stir in Chocó chips.
5. Make cookies from mixture and place on a baking tray.
6. Bake for 10 minutes.
7. Allow to cool completely then serve.

Nutrition: Calories 44 Fat 3.5 g Carbohydrates 2.2 g Sugar 0.1 g Protein 1.5 g Cholesterol 12 mg

473. Pumpkin Pie

Preparation Time: 10 minutes
Servings: 4
Ingredients:
- 3 eggs
- 1/2 cup pumpkin puree
- 1/2 tsp cinnamon
- 1/2 tsp vanilla
- 1/4 cup Swerve
- 1/2 cup cream
- 1/2 cup unsweetened almond milk

Directions:
1. Preheat the oven to 350 F/ 180 C.
2. Spray a square baking dish with cooking spray and set aside.
3. In a large bowl, add all ingredients and whisk until smooth.
4. Pour pie mixture into the dish and bake in preheated oven for 30 minutes.
5. Remove from oven and set aside to cool completely.

6. Place into the refrigerator for 1-2 hours.
7. Cut into the pieces and serve.

Nutrition: Calories 84 Fat 5.5 g Carbohydrates 4.4 g Sugar 1.9 g Protein 4.9 g Cholesterol 128 mg

474. Baked Creamy Custard with Maple

Preparation Time: 10 minutes
Cooking Time: 15 minutes
Servings: 6
Ingredients:
- 2 1/2 cups half-and-half, fat-free
- 1/2 cup egg substitute, cholesterol-free
- 1/4 cup sugar
- 2 teaspoons vanilla
- Dash ground nutmeg
- 3 cups of boiling water
- 2 tablespoons of maple syrup

Directions:
1. Spray 6 ramekins or custard cups with light non-stick cooking spray. Preheat your oven to 325ºF.
2. Combine first five ingredients and mix well. Pour into your ramekins.
3. Pour the boiling water in a 13x9-inch baking dish. Place the ramekins in the dish and bake 1 hour 15 minutes.
4. Cool the ramekins on a cooling rack. Cover with a plastic wrap and chill in the fridge overnight.
5. Drizzle with maple syrup before serving.

Nutrition: Calories: 131 Carbohydrates: 23 g Fiber: 0 g Fats: 1 g Sodium: 139 mg Protein: 5 g

475. Blueberry Yogurt Custard

Preparation Time: 5 minutes
Cooking Time: 15 minutes
Servings: 6
Ingredients:
- 1-6 ounces' container plain yogurt, fat-free
- 2 teaspoons honey
- 1/8 teaspoon of ground nutmeg
- 1/2 cup fresh blueberries (or thawed frozen blueberries)
- 1 tablespoon all fruit blueberry preserves (or raspberry preserves)
- 1 tablespoon toasted sliced almonds

Directions:
1. Drain and thicken yogurt in the fridge using a paper towel lined strainer for 20 minutes.
2. Combine drained yogurt, nutmeg and honey.
3. Combine fruit and preserves; and then spoon over the yogurt. Top with almonds and serve.

Nutrition: Calories: 261 Carbohydrates: 49 g Fiber: 3 g Fats: 3 g Sodium: 137 mg Protein: 11 g

476. Strawberries in Honey Yogurt Dip

Preparation Time: 5 minutes
Cooking Time: 0 minutes
Servings: 4
Ingredients:

- 1 cup plain yogurt, low-fat
- 1 tablespoon of orange juice
- 1 to 2 teaspoons of honey
- Ground cinnamon
- 1 quart of fresh strawberries (remove stems)

Directions:
1. Combine first four ingredients to make a sauce. Pour over strawberries and serve.

Nutrition: Calories: 88 Carbohydrates: 16 g Fiber: 4 g Fats: 1 g Sodium: 41 mg Protein: 4 g Diabetic Exchange: 1/2 Milk, 1 Fruit

477. **Fruit Parfait**

Preparation Time: 10 minutes
Cooking Time: 0 minutes
Servings: 6
Ingredients:

- 1/4 cup sliced strawberries
- 1/2 small sliced peach
- 1/4 cup of fresh raspberries
- 1/4 cup sour cream, fat-free
- 1 tablespoon Blend for Baking Splenda Brown Sugar
- 1/8 teaspoon of almond extract
- Fresh mint for garnish

Directions:
1. In a tall glass, arrange fruits in a layer and set aside.
2. Whisk the remaining ingredients together and pour into the glass. Garnish it with fresh mint.

Nutrition: Calories: 157 Carbohydrates: 33 g Fiber: 3 g Fats: 1 g Sodium: 47 mg Protein: 1 g

478. **Frozen Pineapple Yogurt**

Preparation Time: 5 minutes
Cooking Time: 15 minutes
Servings: 4
Ingredients:

- 1/4 cup egg substitute, cholesterol-free
- 1/4 cup sugar
- 1/2 cup half-and-half, fat-free
- 1/2 cup plain yogurt, reduced-fat
- 3/4 cup of crushed pineapple (keep in juice)

Directions:
1. Beat together the first two ingredients until it thickens and turns cream in color. Add the remaining ingredients and mix well.
2. Chill in the fridge then transfer to an ice cream maker. Follow manufacturer's instructions.
3. Stir and scrape every 10 minutes for an hour while in the ice cream maker or until it turns into your desired consistency.
4. Keep refrigerated.

Nutrition: Calories: 130 Carbohydrates: 25 g Fiber: 1 g Fats: 1 g Sodium: 79 mg Protein: 5 g

479. **Fruity Red Granita**

Preparation Time: 5 minutes
Cooking Time: 15 minutes
Servings: 4
Ingredients:

- 5 cups watermelon, cubed and seeded
- 1/2 cup sugar
- 1 envelope of unflavored gelatin
- 1/2 cup of cranberry juice cocktail

Directions:
1. Pulse watermelon in food processor until nearly smooth.
2. Combine gelatin and sugar and dissolve in cranberry juice over low heat.
3. Add the gelatin mixture in the pureed watermelon and pulse until combined.
4. Transfer to an 8-inch pan, cover and freeze for about 5 hours or until set. Break the watermelon mixture into chunks and freeze again for another 3 hours or until firm.
5. Stir and scrape to create an icy texture before serving.

Nutrition: Calories: 88 Carbohydrates: 22 g Fiber: 1 g Fats: 0 g Sodium: 5 mg Protein: 1 g

480. **Homemade Ice Cream Cake**

Preparation Time: 10minutes
Cooking Time: 15 minutes
Servings: 4
Ingredients:

- 5 sugar cones, crushed
- 3 tablespoons melted unsalted butter
- 4 cups light ice cream, no-sugar-added and softened, divided
- 1-8 ounces' container whipped topping, reduced-fat and frozen thawed

Directions:
1. Grease a deep pie pan dish with cooking spray.
2. Crush sugar cones in a sealed bag using a rolling pin. Place in a bowl. Stir in the butter until evenly moistened. Use the mixture as your crust. Press onto the bottom of the pan and refrigerate for 20 minutes.
3. Layer 2 cups of the light ice cream over the crust and freeze for 30 minutes or until firm.
4. Spread the remaining light ice cream on top of the frozen first layer and freeze again for another 30 minutes.
5. Spread the whip topping on top then freeze for 2 hours or until it is firm.
6. Let ice cream cake soften for 15 to 30 minutes inside the fridge before slicing and serving.

Nutrition: Calories: 118 Carbohydrates: 15 g Fiber: 1 g Fats: 5 g Sodium: 35 mg Protein: 2 g

481. **Almond Strawberry Pastries**

Preparation Time: 5 minutes
Cooking Time: 15 minutes
Servings: 4
Ingredients:

- 12 sheets 14x9-inch phyllo dough
- 1-10 ounces jar strawberry all-fruit spread
- 1/4 cup of slivered almonds

Directions:

1. Layer three sheets of phyllo dough spritzing in between them with cooking spray.
2. Spread a fourth of strawberry within ½-inch of the edges. Sprinkle a fourth of the slivered almonds.
3. Roll the phyllo jelly-roll style starting from a long side. Moisten edges with water to seal. Cut roll into three equal pieces. Repeat to make three more rolls.
4. Arrange 1 inch apart on a greased baking sheet with the cut side down. Spritz the top with cooking spray and bake 12 to 15 minutes at oven temperature of 375ºF or until golden brown.

Nutrition: Calories: 101 Carbohydrates: 19 g Fiber: 1 g Fats: 2 g Sodium: 51 mg Protein: 6 g

482. **Creamy Strawberry Coconut Cones**

Preparation Time: 35 minutes
Cooking Time: 5 minutes
Servings: 4
Ingredients:

- 4 sheets 14x0-inch phyllo dough
- Filling:
- 1 cup cold milk, fat-free
- 1/2 teaspoon of coconut extract
- 1-3.4 ounces package instant pudding mix, vanilla
- 1/3 cup shredded coconut, sweetened finely chopped
- 1/2 cup whipped topping, reduced-fat
- 6 fresh strawberries (leave 3 for garnishing)

Directions:

1. Prepare four pieces 12x6-inch foil and fold half widthwise. Shape each in a loosely rolled cone with edges overlapping by an inch and half.
2. Spray two phyllo sheets with cooking spray and keep remaining covered with plastic wrap and damp towel to prevent drying.
3. Cut in half widthwise and lengthwise and wrap one section on foil cone. Spray with cooking spray.
4. Baked 4 to 5 minutes at 425ºF or until slightly browned.
5. Repeat step 14 process until you make 8 cones.
6. Whisk the first three ingredients of the filling for 2 minutes. Fold in the next two ingredients. Fill a pastry bag with star tip with the pudding mixture.
7. Finely chop three strawberries and distribute between the cones. Pipe pudding into cones.
8. Slice remaining strawberries to use as garnish. Serve immediately.

Nutrition: Calories: 87 Carbohydrates: 16 g Fiber: 1 g Fats: 2 g Sodium: 164 mg Protein: 2 g

483. **Berry Almond Parfait**

Preparation Time: 20 minutes
Cooking Time: 30 minutes
Servings: 4
Ingredients:

- 1-8 ounces' container plain yogurt, low-fat and drained
- 1 cup of sliced strawberries
- 1/2 cup raspberries
- 1/2 cup blueberries
- 1/8 teaspoon of almond extract
- 1 tablespoon pourable sugar substitute + 2 teaspoons, divided
- 2 tablespoons toasted slivered almonds for toppings

Directions:

1. Drain and thicken yogurt in the fridge using a paper towel lined strainer for 2 hours to 24 hours. (Do this the night before).
2. Combine all ingredients but using only 2-teaspoon sugar substitute. Toss lightly to mix. Chill for 30 minutes to 2 hours.
3. Transfer the drained yogurt to a bowl and stir in the remaining sugar substitute.
4. Layer 1/3 cup of berries mixture and half yogurt alternately in 2 parfait glasses.
5. Top with almonds to serve.

Nutrition: Calories: 220 Carbohydrates: 30 g Fiber: 6 g Fats: 6 g Sodium: 84 mg Protein: 9 g

484. **Spice Cake**

Preparation Time: 10 minutes
Cooking Time: 50 minutes
Servings: 10
Ingredients:

- Almond flour: 2 cups
- Erythritol sweetener: ½ cup
- Baking powder: 2 teaspoons
- Ground cinnamon: 1 teaspoon
- Ground ginger: 1 teaspoon
- Ground cloves: ¼ teaspoon
- Salt: ¼ teaspoon
- Eggs: 2
- Butter, unsalted, melted: 1/3 cup
- Water, divided: 1 1/3 cup
- Vanilla extract, unsweetened: ½ teaspoon
- Chopped toasted pecans: 3 tablespoons

Directions:

1. Place all the ingredients in a bowl, reserving 1 cup water and pecans, and stir well using a hand mixer until incorporated and a smooth batter comes together.
2. Take a 7-inch baking pan, spoon the batter on it, then smooth the top, sprinkle with pecans and cover the pan with aluminum foil.
3. Switch on the instant pot, pour in water, insert a trivet stand and place pan on it.
4. Shut the instant pot with its lid in the sealed position, then press the 'cake' button, press '+/-' to set the cooking time to 40 minutes and cook at high-pressure setting; when the pressure builds in the pot, the cooking timer will start.
5. When the instant pot buzzes, press the 'keep warm' button, release pressure naturally for 10 minutes, then do a quick pressure release and open the lid.
6. Take out the pan, uncover it, invert the pan on a plate to take out the cake and let cool for 10 minutes.

7. Spread cream on top of the cake, then cut into slices and serve.

Nutrition: Calories: 229 Fat: 21 g Protein: 6 g Net Carbs: 2 g Fiber: 0 g

485. Chocolate Avocado Ice Cream

Preparation Time: 10 minutes
Cooking Time: 0 minutes
Servings: 6
Ingredients:

- Large organic avocados, pitted: 2
- Erythritol, powdered: ½ cup
- Cocoa powder, organic and unsweetened: ½ cup
- Drops of liquid stevia: 25
- Vanilla extract, unsweetened: 2 teaspoons
- Coconut milk, full-fat and unsweetened: 1 cup
- Heavy whipping cream, full-fat: ½ cup
- Squares of chocolate, unsweetened and chopped: 6

Directions:

1. Scoop out the flesh from each avocado, place it in a bowl and add vanilla, milk, and cream and blend using an immersion blender until smooth and creamy.
2. Add remaining ingredients except for chocolate and mix until well combined and smooth.
3. Fold in chopped chocolate and let the mixture chill in the refrigerator for 8 to 12 hours or until cooled.
4. When ready to serve, let ice cream stand for 30 minutes at room temperature, then process it using an ice cream machine as per manufacturer instruction.
5. Serve immediately.

Nutrition: Calories: 216.7 Fat: 19.4 g Protein: 3.8 g Net Carbs: 3.7 g Fiber: 7.4 g

486. Mocha Mousse

Preparation Time: 35 minutes
Cooking Time: 0 minutes
Servings: 4
Ingredients:

- For the Cream Cheese:
- Cream cheese, softened and full-fat: 8 ounces
- Sour cream, full-fat: 3 tablespoons
- Butter, softened: 2 tablespoons
- Vanilla extract, unsweetened: 1 ½ teaspoons
- Erythritol: 1/3 cup
- Cocoa powder, unsweetened: ¼ cup
- Instant coffee powder: 3 teaspoons
- For the Whipped Cream:
- Heavy whipping cream, full-fat: 2/3 cup
- Erythritol: 1 ½ teaspoon
- Vanilla extract, unsweetened: ½ teaspoon

Directions:

1. Prepare cream cheese mixture: For this, place cream cheese in a bowl, add sour cream and butter then beat until smooth.
2. Now add erythritol, cocoa powder, coffee, and vanilla and blend until incorporated, set aside until required.

3. Prepare whipping cream: For this, place whipping cream in a bowl and beat until soft peaks form.
4. Beat in vanilla and erythritol until stiff peaks form, then add 1/3 of the mixture into cream cheese mixture and fold until just mixed.
5. Then add remaining whipping cream mixture and fold until evenly incorporated.
6. Spoon the mousse into a freezer-proof bowl and place in the refrigerator for 2 ½ hours until set.
7. Serve straight away.

Nutrition: Calories: 421.7 Fat: 42 g Protein: 6 g Net Carbs: 6.5 g Fiber: 2 g

487. Chocolate Muffins

Preparation Time: 10 minutes
Cooking Time: 30 minutes
Servings: 8
Ingredients:

- Pumpkin, chopped, steamed: 2 cups
- Coconut flour: 1/2 cup
- Salt: 1/8 teaspoon
- Erythritol sweetener: 4 tablespoons
- Cacao powder, unsweetened: 1 cup
- Collagen protein powder: 1/2 cup
- Baking soda: 1 teaspoon
- Cacao butter, melted: 4.6 ounces
- Avocado oil: 1/2 cup
- Apple cider vinegar: 2 teaspoons
- Vanilla extract, unsweetened: 3 teaspoons
- Eggs, pastured: 3

Directions:

1. Set oven to 350 degrees F and let preheat until muffins are ready to bake.
2. Add all the ingredients in a food processor or blender, except for collagen, and pulse for 1 to 2 minutes or until well combined and incorporated.
3. Then add collagen and pulse at low speed until just mixed.
4. Take an eight cups silicon muffin tray, grease the cups with avocado oil and then evenly scoop the batter in them.
5. Place the muffin tray into the oven and bake the muffins for 30 minutes or until thoroughly cooked and a knife inserted into each muffin comes out clean.
6. When done, let muffins cool in the pan for 10 minutes, then take them out from the tray and cool on the wire rack.
7. Place muffins in a large freezer bag or wrap each muffin with a foil and store them in the refrigerator for four days or in the freezer for up to 3 months.
8. When ready to serve, microwave muffins for 45 seconds to 1 minute or until thoroughly heated and then serve with coconut cream.

Nutrition: Calories: 111 Fat: 9.9 g Protein: 2.8 g Net Carbs: 3 g Fiber: 1 g

488. Lemon Fat Bombs

Preparation Time: 40 minutes
Cooking Time: 0 minutes

Servings: 10
Ingredients:

- Coconut butter, full-fat: 3/4 cup
- Avocado oil: 1/4 cup
- Lemon juice: 3 tablespoons
- Zest of lemon: 1
- Coconut cream, full-fat: 1 tablespoon
- Erythritol sweetener: 1 tablespoon
- Vanilla extract, unsweetened: 1 teaspoon
- Salt: 1/8 teaspoon

Directions:

1. Place all the ingredients for fat bombs in a blender and pulse until well combined.
2. Take a baking dish, line it with parchment sheet, then transfer the fat bomb mixture on the sheet and place the sheet into the freezer for 45 minutes until firm enough to shape into balls.
3. Then remove the baking sheet from the freezer, roll the fat bomb mixture into ten balls, and arrange the fat bombs on the baking sheet in a single layer.
4. Return the baking sheet into the freezer, let chilled until hard and set, and then store in the freezer for up to 2 months.
5. Serve when required.

Nutrition: Calories: 164 Fat: 16.7 g Protein: 1.3 g Net Carbs: 0.4 g Fiber: 3 g

489. Banana Split Sundae

Preparation Time: 10 minutes
Cooking Time: 0 minutes
Servings: 4
Ingredients:

- 3 frozen, sliced overripe bananas (see Tip)
- 2 tbsps. peanut butter
- 1 tbsp. thawed frozen light whipped topping
- 1 tsp. sugar-free chocolate-flavor syrup
- 1 tsp. chopped peanuts
- 1 maraschino cherry

Directions:

1. Combine peanut butter and bananas in a food processor. Process with cover until almost no lumps remain. Scoop the mixture into sundae dishes.
2. Garnish top with whipped topping, maraschino cherry, peanuts and sugar-free chocolate-flavor syrup. Serve right away.

Nutrition: Calories: 166 calories Total Carbohydrate: 27 g Cholesterol: 0 mg Total Fat: 6 g Fiber: 3 g Protein: 3 g Sodium: 60 mg Sugar: 14 g Saturated Fat: 2 g

490. Berry-lemon Ice Pops

Preparation Time: 15 minutes
Cooking Time: 30 minutes
Servings: 8
Ingredients:

- 1 lemon
- 1½ cups fresh strawberries, quartered
- 1½ cups fresh blueberries
- ¼ cup water

- ¼ cup honey

Directions:

1. Take off 2 tsp. of zest and squeeze 1 tbsp. of juice from the lemon. Mix together the water, blueberries and strawberries in a food processor or blender. Put a cover and process or blend until it becomes almost smooth. Add honey, juice and lemon zest. Put a cover and process or blend until blended.
2. Pour the mixture into eight ice pop molds or 3-oz. paper cups, then insert sticks in the molds. Use foil to cover each cup if you're using paper cups. Slice a small slit in the foil and insert wooden stick into each pop, then let it freeze overnight or until it becomes firm.

Nutrition: Calories: 53 calories Total Carbohydrate: 14 g Total Fat: 0 g Fiber: 1 g Protein: 0 g Sodium: 1 mg Sugar: 12 g Saturated Fat: 0 g

491. Blackberry-banana Lemon Trifles

Preparation Time: 10 minutes
Cooking Time: 10 minutes
Servings: 2
Ingredients:

- 2 3.75-oz. containers lemon sugar-free reduced-calorie ready-to-eat pudding (or use vanilla, with ¼ tsp. lemon zest stirred into each container)
- 1 small banana, sliced
- ½ cup fresh blackberries, blueberries, raspberries or sliced strawberries
- 1 100-calorie pack shortbread cookies, coarsely broken

Directions:

1. Divide a pudding container between 2 straight-sided 8-oz. glasses, evenly spooning the pudding into glasses. Top them with half the banana slices, half the berries, and half the cookie crumbs. Repeat the layers with leftover pudding, banana, berries and cookies.

Nutrition: Calories: 165 calories; Total Carbohydrate: 35 g Cholesterol: 0 mg Total Fat: 3 g Fiber: 3 g Protein: 2 g Sodium: 236 mg Sugar: 11 g Saturated Fat: 2 g

492. Caramel Popcorn

Preparation Time: 30 minutes
Cooking Time: 10 minutes
Servings: 20
Ingredients:

- 1 cup butter
- 2 cups brown sugar
- 1/2 cup corn syrup
- 1 tsp. salt
- 1/2 tsp. baking soda
- 1 tsp. vanilla extract
- 5 quarts popped popcorn

Directions:

1. Start preheating the oven to 250°F (95°C). In a very big bowl, put popcorn.
2. Melt butter over medium heat in a medium-sized saucepan. Mix in salt, corn syrup, and brown sugar.

Boil it, tossing continually. Boil without tossing for 4 minutes. Take away from the heat and mix in vanilla and soda. Add to the popcorn in a thin flow, tossing to blend.

3. Put in 2 big shallow cookie sheets and bake in the preheated oven for 1 hour, tossing every 15 minutes. Take out of the oven and let cool fully and then crumble into chunks.

Nutrition: Calories: 253 calories Total Carbohydrate: 32.8 g Cholesterol: 24 mg Total Fat: 14 g Protein: 0.9 g Sodium: 340 mg

493. **Chocolate-covered Prosecco Strawberries**

Preparation Time: 20 minutes
Cooking Time: 45 minutes
Servings: 2
Ingredients:

- 12 medium strawberries, rinsed and dried
- 2 cups prosecco or other sparkling wine
- ⅓ cup bittersweet chocolate chips (2 oz.)

Directions:

1. In a medium bowl, combine prosecco and strawberries. Keep the strawberries submerged by placing a bowl on top. Cover and place in the refrigerator overnight or for at least 8 hours.

2. Transfer the strawberries to a plate lined with paper towels and pat dry. In a microwave-safe bowl, put the chocolate chips. Microwave in 20-second intervals on High, stirring each interval, until chocolate is melted, about 1 minute. Dip strawberries into the chocolate and put them onto a plate lined with waxed paper. Let sit in refrigerator until the chocolate is firm, about 15 to 20 minutes.

Nutrition: Calories: 50 calories; Total Carbohydrate: 7 g Cholesterol: 0 mg Total Fat: 3 g Fiber: 1 g Protein: 1 g Sodium: 0 mg Sugar: 5 g Saturated Fat: 1 g

494. **Creamy Chocolate Pie Ice Pops**

Preparation Time: 15 minutes
Cooking Time: 15 minutes
Servings: 9
Ingredients:

- 1 (4-serving size) package fat-free, sugar-free, reduced-calorie chocolate instant pudding mix
- 2 cups unsweetened almond milk or fat-free milk
- 1 cup frozen light whipped topping, thawed
- 1 oz. dark chocolate, melted
- 1 tbsp. crushed graham crackers

Directions:

1. Whisk together almond milk and pudding mix for 2 to 3 minutes in a medium bowl or until thick. Fold in whipped topping.

2. Ladle mixture into nine 3-oz. paper cups or ice pop molds. Insert sticks into the molds. In case you're using paper cups, use foil to cover each cup, make a small slit in the foil and then insert a wooden stick into each pop. Freeze overnight or until firm.

3. Unmold the pops. As you work with one pop at a time, drizzle with the melted chocolate and immediately sprinkle with graham crackers.

Nutrition: Calories: 60 calories; Total Carbohydrate: 9 g Cholesterol: 0 mg Total Fat: 3 g Fiber: 1 g Protein: 1 g Sodium: 175 mg Sugar: 2 g Saturated Fat: 2 g

495. **Devil's Food Ice Cream Pie**

Preparation Time: 20 minutes
Cooking Time: 30 minutes
Servings: 12
Ingredients:

- 1 (6.75 oz.) package fat-free devil's food cookie cakes (12 cookies)
- ¼ cup peanut butter
- ¼ cup hot water
- 1 cup sliced bananas
- 4 cups low-fat or light vanilla, chocolate or desired flavor ice cream, softened (see Tip)
- 3 tbsps. fat-free, sugar-free hot fudge ice cream topping

Directions:

1. Chop the cookies coarsely. In the bottom of an 8-inch spring form pan, place the cookie pieces. In a small bowl, whisk together the hot water and peanut butter until it becomes smooth, then drizzle it evenly on top of the cookies.

2. Put slices of banana on top and carefully scoop the ice cream evenly all over. Spread the ice cream until it becomes smooth on top. Use foil or plastic wrap to cover and let it freeze for 8 hours or until it becomes firm.

3. Allow it to stand for 10 minutes at room temperature prior to serving. Take off the sides of the pan, then slice it into wedges. Drizzle the fudge topping on top of the wedges.

Nutrition: Calories: 173 calories; Total Carbohydrate: 33 g Cholesterol: 7 mg Total Fat: 3 g Fiber: 1 g Protein: 4 g Sodium: 90 mg Sugar: 9 g Saturated Fat: 1 g

496. **Fresh-squeezed Pink Lemonade Ice Pops**

Preparation Time: 15 minutes
Cooking Time: 15 minutes
Servings: 7
Ingredients:

- 1¾ cups water
- ¾ cup lemon juice
- ⅓ cup sugar (see Tip)
- Red food coloring (optional)
- Snipped fresh basil or small fresh basil leaves (optional)

Directions:

1. Mix together sugar, lemon juice and water in a 4-cup liquid measure, while stirring, until sugar has dissolved. Tint with food coloring and put in basil, if wanted (it is about to float on top initially).

2. Transfer the mixture into 7 ice pop molds or 3-oz. paper cups. Tuck sticks in the molds. Use foil to cover each cup if you use paper cups; chop a small

slit in foil to tuck in each pop with a wooden stick. Place in the freezer to chill for 1 1/2 hours while shaking molds gently or mixing mixture in cups to disperse basil. Keep on freezing until firm or overnight.

Nutrition: Calories: 43 calories; Total Carbohydrate: 11 g Total Fat: 0 g Fiber: 0 g Protein: 0 g Sodium: 2 mg Sugar: 10 g Saturated Fat: 0 g

497. Han Fro-yo

Preparation Time: 10 minutes
Cooking Time: 10 minutes
Servings: 4

- 3 very ripe bananas
- 1 cup whole-milk vanilla yogurt
- 2 tsps. activated charcoal (see Tip)

Directions:
1. Process activated charcoal, yogurt and bananas till smooth in a food processor; put into medium bowl. Freeze for 5 hours till firm.

Nutrition: Calories: 136 calories Total Carbohydrate: 28 g Cholesterol: 8 mg Total Fat: 2 g Fiber: 2 g Protein: 3 g Sodium: 36 mg Sugar: 19 g Saturated Fat: 1 g

498. Marinated Strawberries

Preparation Time: 15 minutes
Cooking Time: 35 minutes
Servings: 6
Ingredients:

- 4 cups (2 pints) strawberries
- 1 to 2 tbsps. sugar
- 2 tbsps. aged balsamic vinegar
- 2 tbsps. finely shredded fresh mint
- 1 tbsp. lemon juice
- 3 cups low-fat or fat-free vanilla frozen yogurt

Directions:
1. Cut off strawberry stems; cut strawberries in half or into quarters lengthwise if large. Mix together lemon juice, mint, balsamic vinegar, sugar, and strawberries in a medium bowl. Cover and let chill

in the fridge for at least 20 minutes or up to 4 hours.
2. Over scoops of frozen yogurt, spoon the strawberry mixture to serve.

Nutrition: Calories: 166 calories; Total Carbohydrate: 33 g Cholesterol: 10 mg Total Fat: 2 g Protein: 5 g Sodium: 77 mg Saturated Fat: 1 g

499. Pineapple Nice Cream

Preparation Time: 15 minutes
Cooking Time: 15 minutes
Servings: 6
Ingredients:

- 1 16-oz. package frozen pineapple chunks
- 1 cup frozen mango chunks or 1 large mango, peeled, seeded and chopped
- 1 tbsp. lemon juice or lime juice

Directions:
1. In a food processor, process the mango, lemon or lime juice, and pineapple until creamy and smooth. You can add a 1/4 cup of water if the mango is frozen. Serve it immediately if you want to have the best texture.

Nutrition: Calories: 55 calories; Total Carbohydrate: 14 g Cholesterol: 0 mg Total Fat: 0 g Fiber: 2 g Protein: 1 g Sodium: 1 mg Sugar: 11 g Saturated Fat: 0 g

500. Plum & Pistachio Snack

Preparation Time: 5 minutes
Cooking Time: 5 minutes
Servings: 1
Ingredients:

- ¼ cup unsalted dry-roasted pistachios (measured in shell)
- 1 plum

Directions:
1. Hull and serve pistachios together with plum.

Nutrition: Calories: 113 calories; Total Carbohydrate: 12 g Cholesterol: 0 mg Total Fat: 7 g Fiber: 2 g Protein: 4 g Sodium: 1 mg Sugar: 8 g Saturated Fat: 1 g

30-DAY MEAL PLAN

DAY	BREAKFAST	LUNCH	SNACKS	DINNER	DESSERT
1	Granola with Fruits	Classic Mini Meatloaf	Cinnamon Spiced Popcorn	Vegan Cream Soup with Avocado & Zucchini	Pumpkin & Banana Ice Cream
2	Apple & Cinnamon Pancake	Chorizo and Beef Burger	Grilled Peaches	Chinese Tofu Soup	Brûléed Oranges
3	Spinach Scramble	Crispy Brats	Peanut Butter Banana "Ice Cream"	Awesome Chicken Enchilada Soup	Frozen Lemon & Blueberry
4	Breakfast Parfait	Taco-Stuffed Peppers	Mini Apple Oat Muffins	Curried Shrimp & Green Bean Soup	Peanut Butter Choco Chip Cookies
5	Asparagus & Cheese Omelet	Italian Stuffed Bell Peppers	Dark Chocolate Almond Yogurt Cups	Carnitas	Strawberry & Mango Ice Cream
6	Sausage, Egg & Potatoes	Bacon Cheeseburger Casserole	Pumpkin Spice Snack Balls	Cherry Apple Pork	Sparkling Fruit Drink: Diabetic
7	Cucumber & Yogurt	Pulled Pork	Strawberry Lime Pudding	Pork Chops and Cabbage	Tiramisu Shots
8	Yogurt Breakfast Pudding	Baby Back Ribs	Cinnamon Toasted Almonds	Root Beer Pork	Ice Cream Brownie Cake
9	Vegetable Omelet	Bacon-Wrapped Hot Dog	Grain-Free Berry Cobbler	Maple Glazed Pork	Fruit Pizza
10	Almond & Berry Smoothie	Easy Juicy Pork Chops	Whole-Wheat Pumpkin Muffins	Air Fryer Roast Beef	Choco Peppermint Cake
11	Banana & Spinach Smoothie Bowl	Slow-Cooker Chicken Fajita Burritos	Strawberry Salsa	Air Fryer Bacon	Roasted Mango
12	Mixed Berries Smoothie Bowl	Crock Pot Chicken Cacciatore	Garden Wraps	Air Fryer Beef Empanadas	Roasted Plums
13	Bulgur Porridge	Crock-Pot Slow Cooker Chicken & Sweet Potatoes	Party Shrimp	Pork Rind	Figs with Honey & Yogurt
14	Buckwheat Porridge	Crock-Pot Slow Cooker Tex-Mex Chicken	Zucchini Mini Pizzas	Pork Fillets with Serrano Ham	Strawberry Shake
15	Quinoa Porridge	Crock-Pot Slow Cooker Ranch Chicken	Garlic-Sesame Pumpkin Seeds	Pork Fillets with Serrano Ham	Chocolatey Banana Shake
16	Pumpkin Oatmeal	Crock-Pot Buffalo Chicken Dip	Roasted Eggplant Spread	Marinated Loin Potatoes	Fruity Tofu Smoothie

17	Oatmeal Blueberry Pancakes	Crock-Pot Slow Cooker Mulligatawny Soup	Cheese and Zucchini Roulades	Almond Crusted Baked Chili Mahi	Green Fruity Smoothie
18	Tofu Scramble	Greek Chicken	Oatmeal Butterscotch Cookies	Swordfish with Tomato Salsa	Protein Latte
19	Tempeh & Veggie Hash	Polynesian Chicken	Party Spiced Cheese Chips	Salmon & Asparagus	Chocolatey Bean Mousse
20	Tofu & Zucchini Muffins	Coconut Chicken	Asparagus & Chorizo Tray bake	Halibut with Spicy Apricot Sauce	Tofu & Strawberry Mousse
21	Strawberry & Spinach Smoothie	Spicy Lime Chicken	Pumpkin Spiced Almonds	Breaded Chicken with Seed Chips	Tofu & Chia Seed Pudding
22	Quinoa Porridge	Chuck and Veggies	Coco-Macadamia Fat Bombs	Salted Biscuit Pie Turkey Chops	Banana Brownies
23	Millet Porridge	Baked Salmon with Garlic Parmesan Topping	Tzatziki Dip with Cauliflower	Lemon Chicken with Basil	Brown Rice Pudding
24	Bell Pepper Pancakes	Blackened Shrimp	Curry-Roasted Macadamia Nuts	Fried Chicken Tamari and Mustard	Chocó Muffins
25	Sweet Potato Waffles	Cajun Catfish	Sesame Almond Fat Bombs	Breaded Chicken Fillets	Chia Strawberry Pudding
26	Sweet Potato Waffles	Cajun Flounder & Tomatoes	Coconut Chia Pudding	Dry Rub Chicken Wings	Cinnamon Protein Bars
27	Tofu Scramble	Cajun Shrimp & Roasted Vegetables	Chocolate Almond Butter Brownies	Chicken Soup	Chocolate Cake
28	Apple Omelet	Cilantro Lime Grilled Shrimp	Blueberry Popovers	Ginger Chili Broccoli	Raspberry Almond Tart
29	Veggie Frittata	Crab Frittata	Nutty wild Rice Salad	Chicken Wings with Garlic Parmesan	Vanilla Ice Cream
30	Chicken & Sweet Potato Hash	Crunchy Lemon Shrimp	Apricot and Pecan Muffies	Jerk Style Chicken Wings	Fresh Berry Yogurt

CONCLUSION

People often eat a little more salt than their body needs. This excess salt in some people can cause excessive blood pressure. The probability of high blood pressure in diabetics is much higher than in non-diabetics. High blood pressure and diabetes is a dangerous pair. To reduce the amount of salt you take, use less salt when cooking and remove salt from the table. Consume little of canned, canned or salted foods for storage. Prepared soups, freeze-prepared foods and similar foods are usually rich in salt.

Eat less fat, especially less saturated fat. The aim of this proposal is to reduce the risks associated with heart health. High cholesterol levels in the blood; heart attack is one of the factors that invite. Cholesterol is also a type of fat produced in the body and blood cholesterol levels are too high, can block blood vessels. Reducing the fat in our food, especially animal fat, helps lower blood cholesterol.

What should the diabetic patient do to protect his / her heart health?

Fish and chicken white meat, red meat (sheep, beef, etc.) prefer, eat as much lean parts of red meat as possible.

Do not add fat to meat dishes.

Reduce the amount of fat you put into the food, instead of oil, use oil, especially olive oil. Prefer boiling and grilling instead of frying.

Do not eat more than one or two eggs per week.

Do not eat offal (liver, brain, kidney).

Prefer half-fat or non-fat diet milk, the amount of fat in the diet in this way to reduce the amount of salads or meals with the addition of olive oil.

Use margarine instead of butter for breakfast and prefer margarines with a high content of unsaturated fatty acids.

Never use tail oil and inner oil.

Allow less salt to be added when cooking and discontinue the habit of adding salt without tasting the food on your plate.

What is Exchange List?

Food exchange lists are used to help you plan your meals while organizing your nutritional therapy in accordance with your symptoms, socioeconomic and cultural status, and you're eating habits. These lists were created by collecting the nutrients whose energy and nutrient values are equivalent in the same group under the name of "change besin. In the change lists, foods were collected in 7 groups as milk, meat, bread, vegetables, fruit, oil and dried legumes. In each group, the name, practical measure and amount of the substitutable foods were determined. According to your daily energy and nutrient requirement, a certain amount of food is selected from these groups each day, and your nutrition plan is organized, and you can choose from these lists, provided that you do not exceed the number of changes given to each group.

Made in the USA
Monee, IL
26 March 2021